Detox Therapy
Detoxing Should Feel Good Too

K. Akua Gray
Curriculum Development Coordinator
A Life Of Peace Wellness Education Institute, Inc.
Houston, TX

BJK Publishing and Distribution
a DBA of Bojakaz Management, LLC
2017

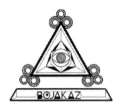

Bojakaz Management, LLC
P O Box 921
Missouri City, Texas 77459
Copyright© 2017 by K. Akua Gray

All rights reserved. No part of this book may be reproduced in any form or by any means including electronic, mechanical or photocopying or stored in a retrieval system without permission in writing from the publisher except by a reviewer who may quote a brief passage to be included in a review.

This publication was designed to provide accurate and authoritative information in regard to the subject matters covered. It is sold with the intention to educate, inform, and empower readers to make their own decisions on health, life, and well-being. If you have concerns about your physical, mental, or spiritual condition consult the appropriate professional.

Cover Design: K. Akua Gray and Cover Fresh Designs
Cover Photo: Anthony Blake
Cover Model: Maati Ra

Printed in the United States of America
ISBN-10: 0-9904089-9-x
ISBN-13: 978-0-9904089-9-4

To Mama and Garry

Also by K. Akua Gray

Naturopathic Reiki I: Opening the Way

☥

Naturopathic Reiki II: The Essentials of Therapy

☥

Naturopathic Reiki III: The Power of the Master

☥

Natural Health and Wellness: The Consultant Manual

☥

Holistic Sexuality: A Practical Guide to Sexual Healing

☥

Today: Wellness Manifestations

☥

Veggie Delights: Holistic Health Recipes, Eating Live for Maximum Nutrition and Wellness

☥

Akwaaba!: Dr. Akua's Ghanaian Vegan Cuisine

☥

Naturopathic Herbology

☥

www.bjkbooks.com

Table of Contents

Introduction	1
Chapter 1 Detox Defined	4
Chapter 2 Toxic Culprits	9
Chapter 3 Time to Detox	39
Chapter 4 The Detox Process	52
Chapter 5 Detox Assessments	55
Chapter 6 Types of Detox	78
Chapter 7 Detox Therapy	121
Chapter 8 Sample Detox Programs	144
Chapter 9 The Detox Therapist Business	161
Acknowledgements	169
About the Author	171
References	172

Introduction

The Detox Therapist is a wellness professional that incorporates every aspect of healing into the process of detoxing including touch therapy, food therapy, spiritual nourishment, emotional balancing and mental changes that will cleanse and purify the whole person with the intention that they will eventually live a life of purification.

To give focus to the body's built-in medicine maker, the immune system, is working hand in hand with the internal and external health faculties to encourage perfect health. When the immune system becomes overloaded, it sends signals throughout the body that it needs detoxing. In natural health and wellness, we focus on the body's ability to self-heal. Sometimes the body needs help depending on the conditions of a person's lifestyle. To become a Detox Therapist is to empower yourself and your clients to trust that built-in medicine maker. Often when the body is off balance with the biochemical restructuring capabilities of synthetically produced medications, the ailment that is being treated can become worse instead of better. That is why in this manual of best health regimens, we will emphasize the ability of the body to heal itself.

The curriculum of Detox Therapy includes identifying how imbalances show themselves through the features of the body, it gives solutions that can assist the body in cleansings, and teaches how to maintain a state of homeostasis through the mental, emotional, physical and spiritual faculties. The body works as a whole system. We have a physical body, a mental body, an emotional body and a spiritual body, and these four bodies work together to make sure that the physical purpose of a person can be obtained, and it also makes sure that all these bodies do their part to assist with living life to the fullest.

It is the physical body that most people think of when it comes to their general health, yet for the majority of people, the body only gets focused attention when it begins to give them problems. It is necessary to make the connection between all the bodies that humans inhabit, including the mental body. The mental body has to do with everything that a person thinks and how those thoughts affect the physical body. The things that we put into our minds also affects the way we live, and when it's time to clean up and release things in life that are not for the individual's greater good, detoxification is only complete when we detox the physical, detox the mind, detox the emotions, and detox the spirit.

These are the components that help to balance and bring equilibrium to the whole person. In Naturopathy, if all these different levels are not addressed in the cleansing process of the client, then the detoxification is not complete.

The body's natural ability to heal itself involves millions of processes that are involuntary and unknown in the presence of daily life. These processes are intended to flow with the order of the natural workings of the human body. This natural rhythm extends the life span of man and allows for what we term as good health for the duration of his time in the physical realm. The fore mentioned in today's world is considered the ideal, because humans unfortunately today live in a world where this ideal natural function of the body has been under assault for more than one hundred years since the onset of the industrial age of the 20th century. Now moving into the 21st century healers can take advantage of the benefit of reaching many people in very short periods of time. This ability makes it easier for therapists to present a program to the masses that communicates the importance of detoxification as a road map to longevity. Detoxification is quickly becoming the way of life for seekers who insist on sustaining purity, maintaining natural protocols for living and elevating their chances of avoiding the vice grip of disease.

Chapter 1 Detox Defined

In Naturopathy, detoxification is the process of moving built up waste/toxins from the body temple. True detoxification means also applying this to the mind, emotions and spirit. To say that a detox regimen is a simple 'cleanse' is an understatement. If this method of healing and regeneration is done properly, it is a restructuring of the physical existence of your client.

Detoxification has been a buzz word in holistic health and mainstream wellness arenas for over five decades. It has become so popular now that every herbal company has a detox product and there are many offerings for detox programs in most wellness arenas. What is going to make you different from all the rest is your level of learning and internalizing the definition of what a detox program really is, as well as the methods of assessments that you will use to assist your clients in seeing how a true detox changes their life. You will use detox as an empowerment tool to change eating habits, release emotional baggage, relieve stress and recondition the mind to put a higher value on life.

We are living in a world where we encounter daily toxins. Take a moment to look around the room that you are in. We live in a chemical culture. This chemical culture is attached to every aspect of the physical world of man: the food industry, home and work products, medications, clothing, transportation and housing. Everything surrounding you for 360 degrees involves chemicals. The paint on the wall, the knobs on the door, the dye in the color of your curtains, the foundation of the mirror on your wall, the dye that's in your sheets, the chemicals that make up your bookshelves, your books, the carpet or the tile on the floor, the ceiling fan and the air conditioning unit that may be cooling the air in your home. All chemicals. We come in to contact with toxins daily and it has become the norm for us. Man has become so accustomed to pollutants and toxins it is not even of a second thought to him until the body reminds him that something in his environment is outside of balance and working against his state of health. No one wants to be diseased or dead. However, the quality of life in today's chemical culture is being reduced. There is a need for educated wellness consultants and therapists who are skilled in the methods of alleviating the premature aging processes, organ degeneration and disease states that exist based on the high levels of chemical intakes within the toxic realm.

The only time we get a little bit of nature is when we step outside of our front doors, and even then, we have to go into the deep depths of nature to breathe a fair amount of oxygen. Most indoor air is only about 20%

oxygen, and because of the pollution in urban areas with dumps that affect the air quality, industrial farm areas that put out greenhouse gases and industrial factory areas, the oxygen level surrounding our homes in the cities and towns are only about 69% oxygen. There are so many things in our environment that we have no control over that affects our bodies on a toxic level.

Although, we do have control over some of the contaminates present in our personal environments, it is unfortunate that many people accept them into their lives for the sake of convenience. That would include items like processed foods, chemical beauty products, deodorants, lotions, makeup and perfumes. In addition to convenience we bring these contaminates into our homes because society has said that in order for the house to be clean you must use a chemical detergent. In order for your body to smell good you must put on a particular perfume, however there is a rule of thumb in detox therapy that we observe, and that is, IF YOU CAN'T EAT IT, YOU SHOULDN'T PUT IT ON YOUR SKIN. Everything that comes in contact with your skin is absorbed into the bloodstream. Therefore, when a person sprays on that perfume designed by the latest celebrity, remember it is not one hundred percent natural, for it may have floral oil in it but mostly it is a chemical agent. The skin is the largest organ of the body and plays a great part in the protection of the body. When unnatural toxic chemicals are absorbed into the blood stream they are recognized by the body as a poison, then the body instantly begins to remove that poison through a process of cleansing. However, sometimes the process of cleansing a saturation of toxins can take time and lead to stagnation, congestion or toxicity in the body.

Another major source of daily contamination is in the foods that are provided by the local supermarkets and food retailers. All conventional farmers, both foreign and domestic use herbicides, pesticides or systemic pesticides. Organic foods are available, but many people choose not to buy organic food because of price or availability. Organic foods can also be home grown, however, very few people dedicate the time to garden their seasonal foods.

Also, in relationship to food, chemical preservatives in processed foods have become a norm in the eating lifestyles of the world. Very few people naturally process their foods any longer, instead it has become convenient to eat solely out of boxes, bags, bottles and cans. Again, people accept this in their lives because the food industry makes it conveniently available.

These contaminants are not new to you, because you live in this world. The question arises, what does it take to live a non-contaminated natural life, and is it possible in today's world? Particularly with our use of cell phones, various gas-powered vehicles and tools that make life a little easier. Some would probably say you would have to go to live in the countryside, grow your own food and live in a naturally designed home. Well that's just about right but very unlikely for those who make their living in the fast-paced urban areas of the world. It is possible to minimize contamination by becoming aware of the options to live life more naturally, and adding a regular detox to any lifestyle will automatically improve life.

Chapter 2 Toxic Culprits

What does a toxic environment look like? There are two levels of toxicity when it comes to environment. The first being the objective. These are the physical things that we experience and therefore affect the human body daily in some way. The second being the subjective, which are the unseen things that we experience when it comes to a toxic environment that affects not only the physical body but the energetic bodies of our existence.

The Objective Culprits

Air pollution is a global problem. The **air quality** throughout the world is being compromised in the name of technology and capitalism which has unleashed extreme pollution often without regard to the safety and the rights of people. Air pollution has become unavoidable. When you breathe you breathe pollution. The majority of air pollution comes from greenhouse gases, factories and vehicles. Think about it. Every city has a factory district that have chemical processing plants and refineries for manufactured goods such as plastic products, beverages, and different types of chemicals and clothing. These factories produce a certain level of pollution in the environment.

Also, cities along the coastal areas have ship channels where cargo ships come into the ports to upload and unload their goods for distribution. I have to admit, I have travelled around the world and I must tell you that the United States has some the best pollution policies that are being implemented. They are really trying. There are some countries that you can go to where they have no pollution laws at all and literally you have to adjust your breath in order to breathe properly or take a few moments to get used to the pollution in the air. Other countries have far worse pollution than the United States.

I would like to visit the Great Wall of China one day however, I have a big hesitation about going to China because of the poor air quality of the country. In China, there are certain days that the government issues warnings to its citizens to forego venturing outside because the air is too hazardous to breathe. On days such as this, people walk around with surgical or oxygen masks. China has become the industrial giant of the world. If you would go around in whatever area you are in and just look at the labels on the different manufactured goods, you'll find about 85% of what you see is "Made in China." Being the largest goods manufacturers of the world comes with a high cost. The Chinese are killing themselves at a fast pace and their government officials and industry leaders have not advanced as rapidly with air cleaning and taking care of the environment.

Here is a short list of the most common air pollutants and chemicals:

Acrolein	Carbon Dioxide
Carbon Monoxide	Nitrogen Dioxide
Nitric Oxide	Sulfur Dioxide
o-Anisaldehyde	Benzene
2, 3 Benzofuran	Coumarin
Formaldehyde	4-Hydroxicoumarin
Menadione	Hydroxyacetophenone
6-Methylcoumarin	6-Methoxytetralone

2-Hydroxy-4-methoxyacetophenone
3-Methyl-2-cyclopentene-2-ol-one
Trimethylbenzene (mixed isomers)
Polynuclear Aromatic Hydrocarbons

Part of your research as a new Detox Therapist is to educate yourself on the nature of these chemicals and pollutants. Become knowledgeable about the effects and conditions associated with these substances in order to communicate this information to your clients where needed.

The **water** ways of the Earth are now dump sites. Companies and individuals continuously desecrate these sacred life-giving portals without regard. As a solution to this, the governments of countries in every part of the world have based their water purification system on the standards of the United States and have created chemical banks in the form of tap water that pours over two hundred disinfecting chemicals into the homes of the world every second of the day to bring in "clear clean water" for bathing, drinking, preparation of food and as a water source to homes. Fortunately, tap water systems do get the water from natural water sources such as local rivers, lakes and springs, however, the treatment process of getting the natural bacteria and the natural parasites out of the water involves an extensive chemical process including chlorinating the water. Local and national agencies say that it is safe for use, however, the body absorbs everything that's put on the skin, even the 200 chemicals that is used in the water treatment systems.

The body is a very resilient organism, but it takes a really big hit when it has to deal with things that are not natural on a consistent basis. The process of aging speeds up and life expectancy decreases. Some people might think that it's ok to die at 65 these days, but it's really not. Not when we know that we have the ability to live well in to the hundreds. Unfortunately, in this chemical culture we find ourselves aging more rapidly than people did in past generations.

We spoke earlier about the chemical content of tap water and this is important because people come into contact with this form of toxicity daily just like the air supply.

As the skin is the largest absorbing organ of the body, to bathe is to submerge oneself into the following:

Acrylamide
Alachlor
Antimony
Arsenic
Asbestos
Atrazine
Barium
Benzene
Benzo(a)pyrene
Beryllium
Bromate
Cadmium
Carbofuran
Carbon tetrachloride
Chloramines
Chlordane
Chlorine
Chlorine dioxide
Chlorite
Chlorobenzene
Chromium
Copper
Cyanide
2,4-Dichlorophenoxyacetic acid
Dalapon
1,2-Dibromo-3-chloropropane
1,2-Dichlorobenzene
1,4-Dichlorobenzene
1,2-Dichloroethane
1,1-Dichloroethylene
1,2-Dichloroethylene(cis)
1,2-Dichloroethylene(trans)
Dichloromethane
1,2-Dichloropropane
Di(2-ethylhexyl)-adipate

Di(2-ethylhexyl)-phthalate
Dinoseb
Diquat
Endothall
Endrin
Epichlorohydrin
Ethylbenzene
Ethylene dibromide (EDB)
Fluoride
Glyphosate
Haloacetic acids (HAA5) (for chlorinated supplies only):
including:
    monochloroacetic acid
    dichloroacetic acid
    trichloroacetic acid
    bromoaceticacid
    dibromoacetic acid
Heptachlor
Heptachlor epoxide
Hexachlorobenzene
Hexachlorocyclopentadiene
Lead
Lindane
Mercury (inorganic)
Methoxychlor
Nitrate (As N)
Nitrate/Nitrite
Nitrite (As N)
Oxamyl (Vydate)
PCBs (Polychlorinated biphenyls)
Pentachlorophenol
Perchlorate
Picloram
Selenium

Simazine
Styrene
2,3,7,8-TCDD (Dioxin)
Tetrachloroethylene
Thallium
Toluene
Total trihalomethanes (for chlorinated supplies only)
  Including: Chloroform
             Chlorodibromomethane
             Bromodichloromethane
Bromoform
Toxaphene
2,4,5-TP (Silvex)
1,2,4-Trichlorobenzene
1,1,1-Trichloroethane
1,1,2-Trichloroethane
Trichloroethylene
Vinyl chloride
Xylenes (total)

Most of the chemicals listed above are intended for water safety, however they are not natural ingredients or natural occurrences in the body. When the body comes into contact with any foreign substances it goes into attack mode to remove the contaminants. Thus, every shower, every bath and every meal prepared with tap water inundates the body with chemicals that the body has to work at removing to reach an optimal functioning level.

If you have heard anything at all about commercial **food** production and distribution in the United States of America and around the world, it probably has not been good. Agricultural chemicals have been used since the beginning of the industrial age. The more people that populate a country, increases the demand for a steady food supply. If you have ever done gardening or farming, you know the insects will wreak havoc on your food supply. Therefore, when farming became big business there had to be a way to harvest foods that were not destroyed by insects. Conventional foods in the markets today are sprayed with various chemicals that include the following short list:

Methyl parathion	Dieldrin
Azoxystrobin	Chlorothalonil
Difenoconazole	Iprodione
Tebuconazole	Trifloxystrobin
Boscalid	Pyraclostrobin
Metalaxyl	Flupicolide
Propamocarb	

There are a million and one things that can be said about the standard American diet and concerns of the food industry. Food has evolved for millenniums and man is still looking for the best ways to maintain an adequate food supply for his prospective regions of the globe. Food has been through splicing, the creation of hybrids, genetic modification, and processing. Many "foods" that people eat today are considered non-foods because by the time it reaches the consumer it may have been through several metamorphoses from its natural state resulting in such products as hot dogs, chips, candy, etc.

The major concerns for natural food advocates and food watch groups is genetically modified organisms (GMO), food chemical contamination and the massive amount of processed foods.

GMO

Genetically modified organisms in food is a laboratory process that involves extracting the genes of an animal or plant and forcing it into a totally different plant. For example, the genes of a fish are forced inside a tomato plant in order to create a longer shelf life for the tomato fruit. According to several consumer reports on food, almost 90 percent of the corn crops produced here in America is genetically modified.

The following is a list of some of the most common genetically modified foods.

1. Corn has been modified to create its own insecticide.
2. Soy has been modified to resist herbicides.
3. Cotton also has been designed to resist pesticides.
4. Papaya has been modified to produce a virus resistant transgenic variety of fruit.
5. Rice has been genetically modified to contain a high amount of vitamin A.
6. Tomatoes have now been genetically engineered for

longer shelf life, preventing them from easily rotting and degrading.
7. Dairy products – It has been discovered that 22 percent of cows in the U.S. were injected with recombinant (genetically modified) bovine growth hormone (rbGH) to artificially force cows to increase their milk production by 15 percent.
8. Potatoes are engineered with Bacillus thuringiensis var. Kurstaki Cry 1 and has toxic repercussions.
9. Peas that are genetically modified have a gene from kidney beans inserted creating a protein that functions as a pesticide.

Credit Source/Article Banoosh - Weblink: http://share.banoosh.com/2012/08/28/top-ten-genetically-modified-foods/#!prettyPhoto-9634/0/

As a healthier alternative to GMO foods, it has been recommended to buy organic foods or grow your own organic foods.

Pesticides, Herbicides and Systemic Contamination

Chemicals used on foods and grown in foods include pesticides, herbicides, and systemic contamination. Herbicides and pesticides are used to keep pest and weeds off the growing foods so that they remain pest free and beautiful for the consumers who will purchase them at the grocery stores. Most people have been eating chemically treated foods all of their lives.

The list of pesticides and herbicides are too numerous to list here, however the food labeling system has made it possible for consumers to choose between two types of produce, conventional and organic.

The food industry created label codes on produce or Price Look Up (PLU) codes, first as a way for grocers to keep count of the foods they were selling with the new digital cash register systems. These numbers were four digit codes beginning with 4. Each type of produce had its own unique number. Later as food advocates began to demand that the consumer be made aware through the PLU which produce were chemically treated, genetically modified or organic, grown with natural to no pesticides, the five digit label code was created.

Label codes with fours are considered conventional which means chemical pesticides and herbicides were used in the growing of that particular item. Produce label codes with an 8 and the four digit code is genetically modified. The last code is the 9 and four digits which denote organic foods. These label codes have become very important for the consumer in order to choose the foods that they are willing to ingest for their health and wellness.

Most grocery stores now give shoppers the choice between the organic and conventional foods. The number of organic farmers and organic foods co-ops have increased over the past two decades throughout the world. Therefore, when you recommend organic foods to your clients they shouldn't have problems finding a retailer or farmer's market with organic foods. Unfortunately, many people have developed a misconception about organic foods being expensive. However, when the price of conventional and organic foods are compared, the price difference is not very significant. For example, fresh kale greens are about $1.49 and a bunch of organic kale about $2.49. Yes, there is a difference but your health is worth it. Your health is worth an extra dollar to buy organic. Also, organic foods are becoming more in demand and major supermarkets are making these foods more affordable. There are no excuses to choose healthy foods, for organic products are readily available. I'll say that if a client is really serious about their health and really serious about having a less toxic lifestyle then organic foods are mandatory. Organic doesn't mean that there are no pesticides or herbicides used. It means that those pesticides and herbicides that are used are natural. An example of a natural pesticide would be a tomato leaf juice spray. The tomato leaves that come on the tomato plant are highly acidic. The solution can be prepared by soaking the leaves in water for an extended period of time, usually about a week. The oxygenation of the leaves causes the solution to become fermented, making it a repellent for most insects. One of the natural pesticides that I also use in organic gardening is neem leaf spray.

I know the coordination and efforts that it takes to change to an organic lifestyle in food consumption. Ideally, growing your own organic foods would ensure healthy eating or buying your produce from local organic farmers which is available in every area of the country, would be best. There are organic farmers at local farmer's markets selling their organic foods and making it affordable to people who want to take care of their health. I grow an organic garden in both my homes, in Houston, TX and Mankessim, Ghana. We also supplement our organic foods by patronizing our local organic farms. In Houston, there are at least a dozen organic coops available each week where local organic farmers gather to sell their fresh produce and organic products. In Ghana, every Tuesday there is an organic farmers market and I travel about an hour up the road. The unique thing about this market is that patrons can either buy or trade their produce, so I take my surplus from my garden for some of the things that I am not growing that other farmers are growing. For myself and my family I have committed to a no excuses policy when it comes to eating organic. I also encourage my clients to make every effort to choose organic foods for best health results.

The most contaminated crops in commercial farming are grown with multiple insecticides and herbicides. According to environmental watch groups, it is highly suggested that if one consumes the following fruits and vegetables, it is best to buy them organic to avoid contamination. The number next to the produce listed below represents the number of chemicals that have been detected in conventional growing.

Peaches (60)
Apples (45)
Pears (36)
Raspberries (50)
Tomatoes (30)
Spinach (50)
Potatoes (30)
Lettuce (50)
Cucumbers (86)

Strawberries (40)
Nectarines (33)
Cherries (50)
Grapes (50)
Celery (60)
Collard greens (45)
Red bell peppers (39)
Sweet peppers (50)

Systemic Pesticides

These are pesticides that are absorbed into the plants tissue during the growth process. Systemic pesticides were introduced into the American food supply in 1998. They are now being more widely used in North America and around the world. The four major types used are:

Imidacloprid is used on tomato and leafy greens.

Thismethoxam is a seed treatment that was first used on corn crops in 2002 and is now used on most vegetable and fruit crops like strawberries and sweet peppers.

Clothianidin which is used as a seed treatment also on rapeseed, "canola," cereal grains, corn, beets and in the soil of potatoes.

> **Dinotefuran** is applied to the soil and sprayed on leafy greens, potatoes and cucumbers.

As an organic gardener, I was first introduced to systemic pesticides at a seed shop in Mankessim, Ghana where I go to the open market for household supplies. In the seed shop I noticed some seeds that looked just like watermelon seeds, but they were blue. I wanted to know why those watermelon seeds were blue. So, I asked the clerk at the counter.

I said, "These are watermelon seeds, right?"
He said, "Yes."
I said, "Why are they blue?"
He said, "Oh it's the chemical. It's good. It will make the watermelons grow big and strong."

I had never seen that before and of course, I didn't get the seeds, but I went back and did my research on the reason for the blue watermelon seeds. I wanted to know exactly what they were doing with the seeds. What I found out was as disturbing as the blue color itself, the agricultural chemical companies spray the pesticide on the seed or they inject the pesticide inside the seed and as the plant grows, it has a time released chemical in it that goes up through the very body of the plant to the flowers and the fruits of the plants in order to repel pests. Systemic pesticides can't be washed off because it is in the biological makeup of the plant and grows within the fruit. I was shocked. I know we are creative people, but we are really creating what is called "franken foods," which are foods that literally are biologically unnatural from the infusion of these systemic pesticides.

Commercial meats are another major source of contamination in the food supply. The chemically produced female hormones DES (diethylstilbestrol) and MGA (melengestrol acetate) are used to induce growth. Nitrate produced meats are also a major source of cancer and disease promotion.

Processed Foods

Poor nutrition is also an objective component of a toxicant environment. People are eating out of boxes, bags, bottles and cans every day. The majority of people in the entire world today do not grow their own foods. Therefore, the past four generations of the world's population have grown to know packaged foods as a way of life. Even when foods are prepared at restaurants, food trucks, and caterers, they also use a majority of their food supplies out boxes, bags, cans and bottles. We call these non-foods because any time real food in its natural form goes through a chemical process or preservatives are added, it turns it into something else. For example, a fruit bar is not all fruit in most cases. It may also contain added chemically extracted nutrients, parts of other substances such as wheat or oils which leaves room for very little of the naturalness of the fruit that it began with.

All processed foods are nutritionally depleted. Any time food is altered from its live natural state through cooking the nutritional value of the food is decreased. Therefore, foods that are in boxes, bottles, can and bags that have been heated do not offer the highest nutrition for consumption.

In nutritional tests on food, broccoli in its live raw state is bright green, vibrant, crunchy and firm, and has a vitamin C rating of 68. When broccoli is cooked it turns a dark mucky green color, it becomes soft, mushy and the vitamin C rating drops to 32. That's more than half of the vitamin C lost in the preparation process of that broccoli. All food is like that, once it is processed, cooked, or heat (pasteurized) treated it becomes less nutritious. Eating cooked and processed food fills the belly, yet often the intake is not nutritionally sufficient to keep the body functioning at its optimal level which can trigger overeating.

Think about your kitchen right know. How many of these foods do you have in your refrigerator or pantry: cow's milk, yoghurt, syrup, jam, jellies, ice-cream, butter, cereals, pies, chips, pastas and breads? Have you fried any of your foods lately? Do you have any processed meat or soy products in your kitchen? These are foods that clog up the immune system and many processed foods create excessive mucus and nervous system stress in the body.

Sugar
Sugar is a major culprit that causes disease in the quest to remain healthy. Most processed foods contain processed sugar. Sugar effects the body in many unhealthy ways. First, when a large amount of sugar is eaten, a paralysis of the immune system occurs. Sugar has chemical components in it that shuts down the immune system for over two hours when the body gets an overload. Let's say a person eats a large piece of cake or a stack of pancakes with syrup for a meal, the excessive amount of sugar paralyzes the immune system cells that fight off bacteria. Think of the parents that give their children the sweet processed cereals in the morning for breakfast and then send them to school to learn. Unfortunately, there is not much learning going on because the concentration level of a child is decreased with the high intake of sugar. Morning meals should begin with a whole grain and plant based protein such as millet, quinoa, oats, wild rice, nuts and dark leafy greens.

A change is in order because the consumer can control certain things, especially food intake when it comes to eliminating toxicity. We don't have to eat cookies. We don't have to eat breads. We don't have to eat cake. We don't have to drink cow's milk. These kinds of products are lifestyle conveniences that have created food and sugar addictions. Concentrated sugar deteriorates the nerves of the nervous system and this aids in the stress on the immune system. It is an addiction to taste, and it creates a toxic environment in the body.

Processed foods have taken another ugly turn recently in a video that has been circulating on social media that was very frightening. There was an Asian chef who had several different bowls of liquids and a large bowl of water. The first liquid was green liquid. He poured a small amount of the green liquid into the water and then all of sudden he started swirling the green liquid around and it started solidifying. He then shaped the green liquid into a small head of what looked like lettuce. Next, he poured some of the red and pink liquid into the water, and when he finished shaping it, it looked like a shrimp. He cut the "lettuce" and "shrimp" in half and put it on a plate and showed it to the camera like "here's your food." I was shocked, but this is what's coming in this chemical culture that we live in. The commercial food industry is making plastic food for people to eat. I looked carefully at the chef's surroundings and the background around him and he was in a kitchen. It is becoming more necessary for people to grow their own food and learn about wild edible plants.

Poverty is also one of those objective factors that breeds a toxic environment. When people are poor, they will often take everything that they can get or whatever is dumped upon them because they don't have the resources to support themselves. There is a movie I would like you to take a look at if you ever get a chance. It's called Darwin's Nightmare. In this movie, you will see how people in poverty are living in a toxic environment surrounding the fishing industry in East Africa. In the documentary, a group of Russians have control of a particular village's fishing industry where the villagers go out and catch the fish. The Russian workers take away all of the good parts of the fish and they leave the scraps, the heads and the bones and the tails for the people. In the fishing village the people are living as if they have no choice but to take the scraps because they consider it good work to work in the factory that filets the fish.

When people live in poverty they don't have quality housing. They live in places that are cheap near factories, dumps and undesirable parts of town. There is a dump in the main town near me in Ghana. Sometimes when I go to the market I have to cross a bridge where you can see the city dump out in the distance, and in that area, there are always people digging around in the dump. I can imagine they are trying to find refuse that they can use for themselves because they have nothing. If you are called to work with those that dwell in poverty it will be necessary to bring forth education and service programs to enrich the lives of the people. The unhealthy habits of poverty are very deeply engrained in the psyche of poor people. In my studies poor sanitation appears to even become a part of some countries traditions, such as open defecation, polluting the water ways, and excessive littering.

Some people also create toxicity in their body by indulging in chemical substances that inebriate and over stimulate the hormonal functions of the body allowing them moments of physical and emotional escapism from the stresses of the world. **Poisonous recreations** such as smoking, drinking alcohol, and recreational drugs are also an objective factor in a toxic environment. People develop habits of smoking tobacco cigars, cigarettes and marijuana. Recently the smoking mechanism that have become popular are hookah pipes and e-cigarettes which are very toxic to ingest and carry the same cancer-causing risk of traditional tobacco products. Going out to bars and getting drunk with friends and coworkers is also considered relaxing and a way to have fun. The long-term effects of these behaviors cause addictions and health problems later in life.

Society and mass media perpetuates these vices daily in most television shows. What is often depicted is somebody taking a drink of alcohol after a hard day's work. The billboard media is continuously saying to the minds of the people that it is OK to get drunk when you want to have fun with your friends. I wrote an article recently on the effects of alcohol. The body actually recognizes alcohol as a poison. When alcohol is consumed, the brain immediately sends a message that a poison is present and begins to constrict the blood vessels to the brain. They close up and provide very little blood supply to the brain. Therefore, when a person gets drunk it's all in the head. They feel woozy, they fall out, they go to sleep and their cognition is impaired. The blood vessels to the brain have constricted in order to protect the body from the poisonous substance . That goes for beer and wine as well. Another thing that happens in the body when a person drinks an excessive amount of alcohol is that they have to urinate because the excretory system becomes activated to begin the process of removing the poison. The body works to release the toxicity through the most rapid means that it can.

For the full article see http://healthy-self-life.blogspot.com/2016/08/have-little-drink-if-you-know-what-i.html

As a detox therapist, you will provide your clients with the help they need to develop a program for the changes they are willing to make. Going through a detoxification process should be a life change. It's not just something to do and then go back to the old way of living. Detoxification should be constant, either seasonally, annually or monthly.

Medications, either prescribed or over the counter (OTC) is a major source of toxicity in the overall body system. Chemical medications are designed to alter the biochemical function of the body. They deplete nutrients in the body and force the body chemistry to be temporarily altered from its natural course so that the medication can complete its purpose. People take medications for a few reasons.

- To mask the symptoms of disease until the body heals itself, i.e. anti-inflammatory medications
- To replace a permanent malfunction in the body, i.e. thyroid medications
- To alter a normal body function to accommodate lifestyle, i.e. contraceptives
- To eliminate foreign agents from the body that disrupt the norm body function, i.e. antibiotics

Long term use of medications can cause an overload of toxic chemical concentrations in the blood. The entire system of blood circulates through the body about every minute depending on the body's activity. With the constant flow of the life force fluid being saturated with a chemical substance, the stress of overload happens very quickly, and people often ignore the signs because they want to keep moving through their busy lives.

Long term use of medications also turns off the body's natural defenses, mechanism for self-healing and fuels dependency on the chemical substance. This creates another biological issue of real physical addiction.

When the person decides of their own free will to stop taking their medications they may experience mild to adverse withdrawal symptoms. If you encounter a client who wants to detox from medications and they make the decision to discontinue their medications themselves, it is wise to advise them to visit their physician or naturopath to assist them with the weaning process.

Another concern from the objective view is with the toxicity of over the counter medications (OTC) which can suppress the body's defense mechanisms. When a person develops a cough, they go get a cough medicine. When they have a fever, they go get a fever medication. When they have a cold, they go get a cold medication. When they have a pain, they get a pain medication. All OTCs are chemicals that cover up symptoms. Understand that when a person coughs, has a runny nose, fever or pain, this is the body's way of defending itself and it shows that the immune system is working. Decongestion medications work against the immune system to stop phlegm from flowing out of the body. Anytime mucus accumulates in the body it is isolating something that's not supposed to be there such as a germ, bacteria, parasite or foreign object. When the mucus starts to come out of the body it is removing whatever it is has isolated that was harmful for the body. Therefore, coughing is a way for the body to isolate and remove substances through the mucus that accumulates in the lungs. That's why grandmother used to say whenever you cough spit it out, because they understood the work of the body and how it defends itself. Coughing helps mucus come out. There is no need to suppress a cough with external medications. The body must be allowed to complete the task at hand.

People use over the counter medications against their immune system because they've been told that if there is a cold, then you are sick, if there is a cough, you are sick and if there is a fever you are sick. When it comes to fevers, even for our little ones, we have been told by the doctors that fevers are very dangerous and the way to treat them is with a fever medication. That is not completely true. When a person gets a fever, again, it is the body's defense mechanism assisting the body in burning off something that should not be there whether it's a parasite, virus, bacteria or germ. Any kind of ailment that the immune system encounters it activates the body temperature system in order to burn it off. If a person was to let a fever run its course usually in a healthy person a fever is over within twenty-four hours. For example, if a child got a fever at two o'clock in the afternoon and parents took the natural precautions of making sure that their body stayed cool, like giving them some lemon water to drink, allowing the child to rest and providing light meals to eat, such as vegetable broth, the fever would more than likely be gone by morning or afternoon of the next day. From a naturopathic point of view, fevers above 104° are considered dangerous, therefore we apply antipyretics which are natural fever medicines of herbology to help keep the fever a little bit lower, but still allowing the body's immune system to not be suppressed with chemical medications.

There are a million and one medications in the prescription marketplace and the pharmaceutical companies are creating new ones every day. Chemical medications are prescribed for everything. It's very interesting how the prescription process works, when medical doctors will write medication prescriptions for everything. Unfortunately, medicines from the pharmaceutical companies are chemically produced which comes which comes with an unhealthy level of toxicity and side effects. It is safer to care for the body by natural means, and the less chemicals, the better. There are some people who need chemical medication to stay alive because they have contracted or been afflicted with an incurable disease. It is unfortunate that many people on lifelong medications are suffering from preventable disease too. This is where the detox therapist comes in as a vital resource to community health with your knowledge of disease prevention and assisting clients with a detoxification process to relieve the body from the stress of the chemical medication component. There are annual reference guides on medications that are good to view in your expanded research from this course, The Physician's Desk Reference and The Pill Book, both can be found in your local library.

We have talked about the objective aspect of the chemical culture and the many physical dangers that we face every day. Now let's turn to the spiritual imbalances such as negative thoughts that also can affect a person's livelihood and is a part of the detoxification process.

The Subjective Culprits

Negative thinking and interacting with each other negatively runs deep in the social make up of people worldwide. Anytime you turn on the television somebody is displeased with somebody about something. There is always some kind of negativity being expressed among people, and that's unhealthy. We are inundated with negative thinking and that is sometimes a result of what we experience in childhood and in the many relationships a person has along life's journey. As a Detox Therapist, you can help clients to detoxify their mind and get out of negative thought patterns. Many of the therapies that we will explore in later chapters will help you to formulate wholistic detox programs that have been proven effective for every aspect of the client, physical, mental, emotional and spiritual.

Dealing with the **emotional drama** of life has people on edge because there is always something going on that's stressful or there is always someone who is upset. Many people just don't know how to live in peace, which makes emotional stress one of those unsafe components that creates a toxic environment. For example, some people smoke cigarettes to calm their emotions and relax their minds, but turning to a toxic substance to relax defeats the cry for help.

Ignorance is also a subjective factor in living a toxic life. For example, there are some people who still smoke around their children. However, since the dangers of smoking have been proven to be a great risk to health there are now new laws being passed to protect non-smokers from this unhealthy method of stress relief. There is a law that was recently passed in Texas, which says parents can no longer smoke in their cars when their children are in the cars. If a person is found smoking in the car with their children, they can be fined for endangering their child's health. When a smoker doesn't know about the law and they are still doing it, then that's considered ignorance. It's ignorance to not know or care that your second-hand smoke affects your child's health. We've all heard stories of people dying or being diagnosed with lung cancer, lung ailments or respiratory diseases but they never smoked in their life, and it's because they were always around a smoky environment.

Are you around someone who gossips all the time, puts down other people, or talks down to you? If so, this would be considered a **dysfunctional relationship**. Relationships that are not nurturing and supportive of your purpose or if you are around someone who is angry and frustrated all the time is detrimental to a healthy lifestyle. When all a person hears is negative thoughts, it programs the brain cells to reproduce a similar vibrational chemistry to the other cells in the body. Dysfunctional relationships, guilty relationships, abusive relationships, all create a toxic environment.

Dysfunctional community is also another culprit in the subjective toxic environment. In Chicago, Illinois for a number of years there have been reports of multiple community shootings almost on a daily basis. Many of the victims in these killings have been children, teenagers, and elderly people who get caught in the crossfire of gang, and rage violence. This type of dysfunction in the community breeds fear and fear creates physical ailments.

An **overburdening work environment** can be a great cause of stress and because people have to work they tolerate features of a toxic work environment such as the gossip, bad vibes and verbal abuse. The issue with stress as a "toxin" is when the person allows the stress levels in their life to mount up to physical, emotional, mental and spiritual disease states.

Stress is an interesting toxin, because although stress can be good for the body in low levels, if the body is burdened with too much stress it can slow down the detoxification enzymes of the liver. **When the body is stressed, its systems often come to a halt.** Stress can make us sick with symptoms such as hair loss, acne, indigestion, constipation, fatigue and pain. Stress is also a biochemical function of the body. When the body encounters stimuli, the brain releases hormones and neurological impulses that helps the body to process first the emotional response, second the physical response and third the mental response to come back into balance.

Detoxification is also important for the mental and emotional health of a person too. Everybody who is living in this world today should have a regular detox regimen. That involves being able to disconnect, regenerate, and flush out. Detoxification also involves letting go of imbalances.

Chapter 3 Time to Detox

Eating Lifestyle and Pollution Exposure

I live bi-continental, usually two seasons in Ghana West Africa and two seasons in the United States. I find that each environment with the different climates and environmental settings require two different ways of caring for my body with regular detox. I do a seasonal detox in the United States and an annual detox when I'm in home in Ghana. I eat a healthy organic mostly raw vegan lifestyle, but I find that my metabolism slows down in the United States and speeds up in Ghana. The two environments are totally different. In the United States, I live in a city that has what we would consider normal rates of pollution based on environmental protection standards of, therefore a seasonal detox is good because I know that I am exposed to far more chemical substances in the air than I am at home in Ghana where I live by the sea in a country village that has no factories and the car to human ratio is about 1:500. Actually, no one in my village owns a car which lessens the pollution levels. Also, in Ghana I grow my own organic foods and can live by the health philosophy of growing what I eat and only eating what I grow, however, in the United States I depend on other local farmers and the health food markets for what I trust to be organic fresh produce.

You will encounter many different clients with various lifestyles and levels of awareness when it comes to being healthy. A **monthly detox** would be for those people that are still indulging in the addictive vices we talked about in Chapter 2, high emotional and mental stress levels and those who have a poor eating lifestyle, or those exposed to moderate and high levels of environmental toxins.

After travelling is also another good time to detox, especially when travelling from one time zone to another at very fast rates by car, train or plane. Let's say for instance when I fly home to Ghana from the United States, that's a ten to fourteen hour flight across the ocean depending on the airline. Now, just imagine for a moment if there was no plane how long would it take me the get there? Ideally based on what history tells us if we would travel in a boat it would take 3 to 4 months. If we could travel on land and walk from the United States to Africa through Russia it would take years, possibly even decades to walk. Thank goodness for modern transportation. However, to get from one part of the world to another in such a short period of time completely throws the body's rhythm off and most people experience jet lag. The most stressful part about this type of time travel is its effect on the organs which have to adjust to the new time because the body is not sleeping when it should be sleeping, and the body is expending energy at an abnormal time. This is an especially difficult adjustment for the digestive system. Another reason that detoxing is good after travelling is due to the poor quality of recycled air at high altitudes in plane travel. The vital organs can become stressed and deprived of oxygen. According to Robert Davis in his USA Today article entitled, "Do Passengers Get Enough Oxygen?" he states:

> "As the plane soars, extremely hot air is drawn from the jet's engines, cooled and piped into the cabin. This constant flow of very dry air keeps a life-sustaining pressure in the cabin. But because the plane is designed to be as lightweight as possible, it can only withstand so much pressure. The thin aluminum shell of most jets expands like a balloon — as much as an inch — as the pressure inside increases and the outside pressure decreases at high altitudes.
>
> There is just as much oxygen in the cabin air at cruising altitude as on the ground, but because the atmospheric pressure is lower than at sea level, it is more difficult for the body to absorb the vital gas. With less pressure, fewer oxygen molecules cross the membranes in the lungs and reach the bloodstream.
>
> The result is a significant drop in the amount of oxygen in the blood — anywhere from 5% to 20% depending on the person, the plane and the length of the flight. With less oxygen in the bloodstream, the vital organs soon get deprived.
>
> The reduced oxygen supply to the brain is why some suffer headaches while in flight, one of the symptoms of hypoxia. When oxygen levels fall in the brain, the heart tries to compensate by beating harder and faster. Another symptom of hypoxia is fatigue."

When I first moved to Ghana in 2009 I would take annual trips to the United States to visit family, and each time I made the long flight, I found myself needing to readjust my respiratory and digestive systems. I would accumulate excessive mucus and my digestive system would show signs of blockage for a few days. This made me realize the importance of detoxing after travelling, even if the trip is simply going from the west coast to the east coast of the United States, for that 3 hour time difference going from California to New York can affect the body systems.

Whenever a person is in a **toxic environment** for an extended period of time it is a good time to detox. Toxic environments are so numerous in the world today that it would take a whole book to list them all, so by definition, we consider **anything that is a consistent obstacle to balance in life creates a toxic environment,** this can be anything physical, mental, emotional and spiritual such as work related stress, difficult relationships, guilt and depression caused by religious beliefs.

Whenever **disease** is present, it is time to detox. Disease is a consistent and progressive system of low energy that causes malfunctions and deterioration in the body. There are nearly forty-thousand classified diseases in pathology, however, most of these diseases cannot thrive in a healthy well-nourished body. Disease progression can be measured on four levels: mild, severe, chronic and degenerative. Knowledge of these levels are important for you as a Detox Therapist because they will help you determine the length of the detox program that you will work with your client on. Mild disease progression would not warrant as long of a detox program as severe, chronic or degenerative, which would be the lengthiest detox regimen.

Organ System Stress

All the body systems work in a process called synergy, where all systems, organs, tissues and cells perform their job in synchrony for the greater good of the entire body temple. There are three ways that organ system stress shows up in the body and that is through congestion, stagnation and toxicity. Symptoms occur in the area where stagnation (no movement), congestion (slow movement) or toxicity (biochemical build up) damage has occurred.

Stagnation is when certain aspects of the body systems and channels stop moving. Constipation, back ache, kidney stones, sexual dysfunction and heart burn are signs of stagnation.

Congestion appears when the body's systems and channels are moving slowly. Obesity, heart disease, acne, menstrual problems, wheezing, and boils are examples of congestion.

Toxicity is when the biochemical process of a tissue, organ or fluid system in the body is contaminated. Such as infection, cancers, drug addictions and allergies. In the client assessment, as therapists we are taught to identify when it's time to detox by surveying the respiratory, gastrointestinal, integumentary, (the skin) urinary, and immune systems. All of these areas are necessary for us to be able to help a person reestablish health through the detoxification process.

The organs that are vital in the detoxification process are the liver, colon, lungs, kidneys and skin. They work to eliminate toxins and waste from the body through the rectum, urinary tract, the mouth and nose (the breath) and pores. Organs can become stressed physically through poor nourishment, disease, emotional stress and addictions. The organs replace the cells in their tissues constantly, however, when the organs are faced with a rapid assault such as a break down in the quality of the immune system and its ability to produce a resistance to an invader, stress can occur which can result in the body signaling the brain that there is something wrong. Since all of the body systems are connected and work together, there is no need to try and isolate a particular organ for cleansing during detox. Instead, it is suggested to focus on the entire body to assist with creating synergy.

One of the key detoxification organs in the body is the **liver**. The liver is the largest organ in the human body and the main source of heat for the body. It is located below the diaphragm in the thoracic region of the abdomen. The liver has many functions including decomposition of red blood cells, protein synthesis, stores water soluble vitamins A, D, E, and K, emulsifies fats and lipids, produces bile, an alkaline compound which aids in digestion, and stores glycogen. Glycogen is a polysaccharide that converts glucose for energy.

The liver protects itself and defends the body against impurities. The liver is the most toxic organ in the body. Never eat the liver of any animal.

True detoxification from a naturopathic point of view is detoxing of the mind, emotions, and spirit, as well as the body. Detoxing the emotions is not a common subject but it should be. One of the things that you will assist your clients with is being able to let go of things that do not serve them in their health goals. Did you know that if a person has different types of excessive emotional stress they can damage their physical body? For example, if a person is angry, frustrated, irritable, jealous, and obsessive they can physically affect the liver's ability to do its job. The liver is such a durable organ. Many ailments of the liver are not detected until they have become chronic. Some symptoms of liver stress include yellow eyes and skin (jaundice), nausea, abdominal pain and swelling.

The large intestine also known as the **colon** collects and stores the waste products from digestion. It is a long muscular tube that pushes undigested food towards the anus for elimination. Undigested food mixes with mucus and bacteria residing in the colon. As the waste moves along in the colon the water is reabsorbed into the bloodstream, and the feces start to solidify. The colon is divided into the following parts: the cecum, the ascending colon, the transverse colon, the descending colon, the sigmoid colon, the rectum and the anus.

There are numerous physical conditions that can affect the colon such as cancer and inflammatory bowels, however, constipation and diarrhea are the most common of all ailments. The colon can also be affected by the emotional health of a person. When there is an overwhelming amount of consistent anxiety and nervous stress, the colon can become constricted.

The **lungs** are the paired spongy respiratory organs situated inside the rib cage that transfer oxygen into the blood and remove carbon dioxide and other waste. With each breath that a person takes, more than one and a half pints of blood in the lungs are directly exposed to the air and toxins that are present. The lungs are equipped with a defense mechanism called a cough. Anytime the lungs become overwhelmed, the immediate response is to clear the lungs. Stagnation and congestion can occur in the respiratory system. Imbalances include labored breathing, coughing and wheezing when the respiratory system needs to be cleansed. The respiratory system operates at its optimal functioning level between three and five o'clock in the morning, whereas deep respiration is a vital part of the body's cleansing and regenerative process that occurs every evening with sleep. That's why sometimes a person may wake up in the early hours of the morning coughing from the cleansing work. This cleansing process is also why when we sleep we automatically breathe deeply.

Mucus, infectious fluids and solid waste particles are expelled from the lungs during detox through breath therapy and purification. It helps with the detoxing process when a person can expand shallow breathing and achieve full deep breathing. Through the detox therapy work you will find some people just need to breathe on all levels, mental, emotional, physical and spiritual. Emotional stress to the lungs can be brought on by worry, grief and sorrow.

We excrete nitrogenous wastes via the **kidneys** which are located on either side of the spine, just under the bottom ribs. They are well supplied with blood via the renal artery and renal vein. Urine made in the kidney collects in the renal pelvis, then flows down the ureter, to the bladder where it is stored until voided.

The kidneys control the quantity and quality of fluids within the body. They also produce hormones and vitamins that direct cell activities in many organs; the hormone renin, for example, helps control blood pressure. When the kidneys are not working properly, waste products and fluid can build up to dangerous levels, creating a life-threatening situation. Among the important substances the kidneys help to control are sodium, potassium, chloride, bicarbonate HCO3 (measured directly as CO2), pH, calcium, phosphate, and magnesium. The kidneys are part of the excretory system that helps flush out the uric acid, excess vitamins, minerals and fat.

The kidneys are very fragile organs. There are over three hundred known kidney diseases including kombucha tea toxicity. Among the detox organs, the kidneys tend to malfunction and deteriorate faster. Diseased kidneys often need to be removed or they need assistance to remain functional with artificial cleansing treatments like dialysis. The emotions again play a vital role in the health of the kidneys, excessive amounts of fear, anxiety and confusion are unhealthy and can also be damaging.

The **skin** is the external protective membrane or covering of the body, consisting of the dermis and epidermis and often covered in hair. Noted as the largest organ of the body, the skin is a major outlet in the detox process. The skin in very close proximity to the lymphatic system will show various signs of imbalances and disease through dryness, pimples, boils, discoloration, changes in texture and a diseased appearance.

The enzymes and melanin hormones in the body are excellent announcers and protectors when it comes to symptom manifestations. As a defense mechanism, both will begin to accumulate in the affected area until the healing agents of the body have completed their work. Sweating is a great companion to detox, it opens the pores to manage the extra heat of exercising and increased activity.

Although the **heart** is a muscle, it too has its role in the detoxification process. The heart is very important in the detoxification process because the heart keeps the body's circulation and the lymphatic system in rhythm.

The heart is affected by the negative emotions of sadness, depression, despair and despondence. These lingering emotions cause hormonal saturation of the cells and most people are unable to function well in life when they are over burdened with trance inducing emotions. This also increases the level of toxicity in their blood which makes the heart have to work harder to reduce said levels. Anytime a person is dealing with excessive emotions they are damaging the heart.

What do we know about emotions and spirit and the mind and spirit? We know that in every part of life including detox time, they all work hand in hand. If the emotions are not right the mind is not going to be right. If the mind is not right the spirit is not at rest.

The natural state of being for all people is a state of peace. Our natural state of being is not happiness. Happiness is an emotion. If the body is ill the mind is not peaceful. If the body is ill the emotions are in a state of fear. If the body is ill the spirit is not at rest because it is the spiritual imbalance that creates the physical manifestation. As a part of universal law, the unseen always happens before the seen.

It is also important to understand the role of the body systems and how they all work together in detoxing. The number one body system that deals with the detoxification process is the digestive system. Colon therapists often say, "Death begins in the colon." There is some truth to that, because if the digestive system gets clear then that will help the other systems of the body begin to work better. Most detoxing processes will start with a digestive system purge such as colon therapy, enemas (self-administered) or an internal herbal purge. The digestive system does help to jumpstart the detox process especially in clients who have large swollen bellies from fecal impaction.

The circulatory system housing the veins and arteries is another area that can become congested, stagnate or toxic. There is such a thing as people having bad blood, "bad" meaning it is not supplying the nutrition that the body needs to function at its optimal level. The arteries supply the oxygen rich blood to the system, which transports all the good nutrients, fluids, and antibodies out to the body. The veins are the disposal aspect of the circulatory system where the toxins, carbon dioxide, viruses, bacteria, excessive fluids and parasites get flushed from the body. The circulatory system helps the kidneys and blood to detoxify.

The lymphatic system can display signs of stagnation, congestion and toxicity. When the client has a cough or mucus drainage, the lymphatic system has isolated something that needs to be released from the body. Sometimes a person will develop boils that show up under the arms, in the groin area and along the neck, these types of boils are not only signs of infection but are actually the lymphatic system working to protect the body through the immune system function. It is a natural process for infection to be released from the body.

Detox therapy is unadvisable with, ulcerative colitis, during pregnancy and breastfeeding, after any major surgery, when post-operative areas are still tender, if a person is weak and unable to walk (non-ambulatory), or when multiple physical complications are present, and when the client is under a medical or naturopathic doctor's care.

Chapter 4 The Detox Process

Any detox program that is less than seven days is not a detox. It is simply a flush or a jump start to the detox process. For the body to undergo a serious reversal of the chemical culture at least twenty-one days is necessary to affect changes in personality, eating habits, home restructuring, relationship restructuring and thought pattern changes that will assist the individual for life. The general steps will involve releasing present blockages, regenerating the flow of the body systems and toning the organs and the tissues.

Release of Blockages

The natural detox process addresses the needs of all the cells in the body. Detoxing improves the circulation of the blood and the ability of the blood to supply nutrients to the tissues, organs and systems. Detoxing is a gradual process and in every healthy lifestyle, ideally, it should be a consistent health regimen.

The first component of detox is to **release blockages** caused by congestion, stagnation and toxicity. It is recommended to begin the detox process from the bottom up. This can be organ system specific. For example, reestablishing the free flow of the digestive system. Once you learned how to identify which organs are under the most stress, you can begin to formulate the best detoxification process for your client. The point is to begin to promote movement with filtering and cleansing by increasing the oxygen and hydrogen levels. This can be done with a regimen of hydration and chlorophyll. Chlorophyll is instant nourishment to the red blood cells. As a nutritional supplement it oxygenates the blood for better circulation.

The body is about seventy percent water with two components of hydrogen and one component of oxygen. I often ask my clients the question, if the body is seventy percent water why are we not consuming seventy percent liquids? This question was designed to get the client to think about what their bodies are and how best to take care of their water body even after the detoxification process is done and the healthy lifestyle begins.

Another very important module to the detoxification process is to give attention to the **pH (potential for hydrogen)**. In layman's term, the pH is how much water is available for the full functioning of the body systems. Once the pH of the body is identified, we are then able to suggest nutrition that will maintain a normal pH to avoid high levels of acid in the tissues caused by poor diet, toxicity and chemical medications which can create malfunctions in all of the organs and systems. The potential for hydrogen measures the pureness of the body's fluids. When the body is

filtering and cleansing well it is healthy. This method of purification is often achieved with nutritional changes.

Regeneration and Toning

Once the organs and systems have gone through cleansing, the body will automatically begin the regenerative and toning process. This part of the detox process involves therapy, nutrition, toning agents and rest. Consistency in these areas will facilitate lifestyle changes. Lifestyle changes should encompass healthy eating, consistent movement, and conscious care of the body. It is only through lifestyle changes that a regular detox has the greatest effect on lifelong health.

Detoxification is not a quick fix. It is intended to be a lifestyle program of consistency to combat the unhealthy ways of the world today. Professional detox services include weight loss, disease prevention, reversing premature aging, faster healing, organ regeneration and detox therapies to condition the body for change.

Chapter 5 Detox Assessments

When does the body need detoxing? There are several common signs including digestive system problems, being overweight or underweight, seasonal allergies, frequent infections, fatigue, headaches, skin irritations, bloated abdomen, menstrual difficulties, unclear thoughts and swelling in the body especially in the face. Other signs include uncontrollable cravings, poor immune system function, depression and anxiety. The list goes on, however, if we refer to the definition of detox, valid obstacles will manifest themselves.

As a Detox Therapist, it is advised that you program yourself to evaluate your client on multiple levels. The physical level will be the first component assessment. This is what you see or what the client tells you is their physical concern. However, what's going on in the client's mind also might be a cause of stagnation and congestion especially if there is negative thinking or self-defeating thoughts at work. What's going on with the client in their emotional state by dwelling on unhealthy emotions about things that are happening in life, or in their relationships also creates stagnation and congestion. Do they find life worth living? Do they live in peace? How is the client living in terms of their spiritual health? These are questions that will be addressed in every assessment.

When body stress manifests it will show up as organ stress first through the face and to confirm this stress we also look at the biochemical health of the body through pH testing and urine analysis. Let's take a look at our clients using some traditional naturopath assessment skills to learn how to identify where the stress is happening in the body. These assessments provide the best way to recommend a detox process for our clients.

Your detox assessment will start as soon as your client walks through the door. The body tells everything through physical and biochemical assessments. There is also a survey and written assessment that will help you gather the information needed to prepare a unique detox program for your client. A Detox Therapist does not diagnose disease, an exclusive right for licensed medical professionals only. Instead, the Certified Detox Therapist uses proven methods of assessment to identify areas of imbalances that the body naturally exposes when it is under stress.

Facial Analysis

I love facial analysis as the results surprises the client every time I use it. The facial analysis that we use in Naturopathy comes from the Ayurveda methods of natural health techniques which has been around thousands of years, making its journey through Africa, Asia, Europe and now here in the United States. The creator sealed up the body with specific openings for specific reasons to ensure survival. This body was designed to serve us for all the days we live throughout the aging process. It was not meant for the body to be cut open, which often causes many complications and at times death. In natural assessment, we use the nerve endings that is relative to the different organs that show up on every part of the body. When we look at the face we are looking at the entire body. With facial analysis, you are able to look at your client's face to see where different areas of stress are present in the body.

The face is divided into three sections. In the upper part of the face the nerve endings of the nervous system are most prevalent. In the middle part of the face the circulatory and respiratory systems manifest, with the lower part representing the digestive and reproductive systems. There are also specific areas of the face with nerve endings to the detox organs, the lungs, liver, and kidneys, as well as other organs like the stomach, gall bladder, spleen and heart. The way to identify any imbalances on the face is through stress indicators. These are specific visuals signs on the face such as blemishes, discoloration, bumps, puffiness, and any alterations in the configuration of the face from its normal structure.

Working our way from the top down, let's take a look at various signs of the face. **Nervous system** stress is evident when the forehead of the client has various lines, pimples or discoloration.

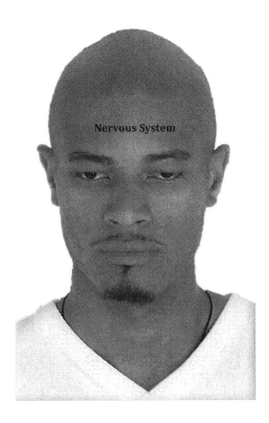

These same indicators can show up on the middle section of the face from the eyebrows to the jawline when there is respiratory and circulatory system stress. At the top of the middle section of the face in the eyebrow and upper eyelids area is where liver and gall bladder stress will manifest. **Liver** stress indicators include puffiness, swelling, or vertical lines between the eyebrows and or darkening of the upper eyelids. **Gall bladder** stress will manifest as a bumpy greasy eyebrow ridge or as bags in the interior corners of the upper eyelids.

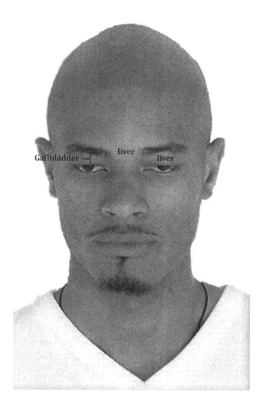

Around the rest of the eye area is where **kidney** stress becomes evident. The kidney stress can be identified very easily as swollen bags under the eyes, darkness around the eyes and crow's feet in the corner of the eyes, which are small wrinkles between the eyes and the temples. The **bladder,** which works closely with the kidneys, also has a facial indicator and manifest as darkness around the lower face and around the mouth.

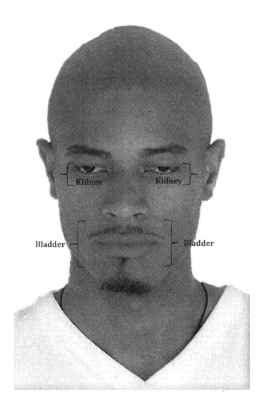

Indicators of **lung** stress include sunken cheeks which indicates poor oxygenation. That means the person's breath pattern is not supplying enough oxygenation from an excessive acidic pH usually caused by smoking or environmental contaminates. Red swollen cheeks indicate mucus or fluid deposits in the lungs, usually from a high intake of dairy foods or not enough physical movement.

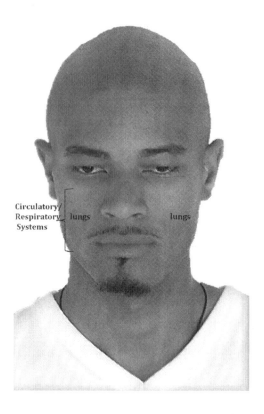

Heart stress can be detected by a red nose, swollen nose or excessive lumps and bumps on the nose.

The lower area of the face begins underneath the nose and runs down around the mouth and ends at the jaw bone encircling the chin. In this area of the face is where digestive system stress manifest in organs such as the stomach, small intestine, and colon. **Stomach** stress has a unique presentation in the upper lip that is usually manifested in people who drink alcohol regularly. The upper lip swells and has a ballooned glossy look which is an indication of an expanded stomach. Another stomach stress indicator is a white colored border around the upper lip which signifies possible indigestion.

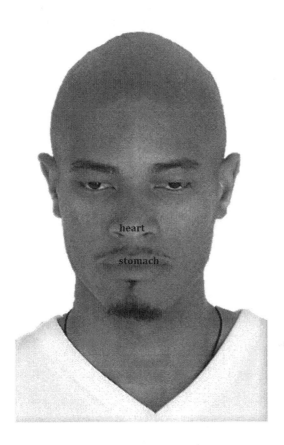

Colon indicators show up as rounded puffiness underneath the corners of the outer lips and tightness of the lower lip as a sign of constipation. Poor absorption in the **small intestine** will manifest as swelling in the central part of the lips.

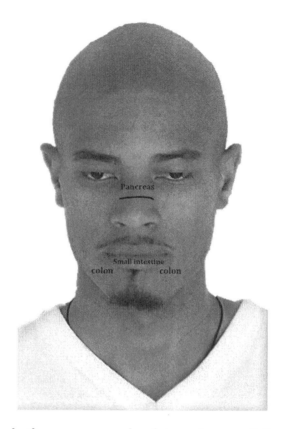

Although the pancreas gland is not one of the detox organs, it does have a significant role in the digestive system and it has a distinct indicator across the bridge of the nose. If there is a dark to black straight line across the nose it shows pancreas stress that may be associated with a hyperglycemia.

The pH (potential for hydrogen)

Measuring the pH of a client will provide you with two very important results that will help formulate a personalized detox program. Testing the pH reveals the biochemical balance in the body, which can be either alkaline or acidic. The other pH assessment result which measures the state of disease progression can help the therapist determine the time necessary to provide an adequate detox regimen.

All organs and tissues in the body have individual pH levels as well. Alkaline pH can be found in the brain, lungs, testes, ovaries, stomach lining, uterus lining, eyes, penis, vagina, breast, liver, fat, capillaries, muscle, diaphragm, skin, and spleen to name a few.

Neutral pH organs and tissue are arteries, veins, hair, kidney, pancreas, intestinal walls, thyroid, esophagus, heart, skin of palms, soles of feet, knee caps, ligaments, cartilage, nails and teeth.

Acid pH organs and tissue are bones and the stomach.

The alkaline and acid balance in the body should be about 80% alkaline and 20% acid. This balance will give a reading of normal on the pH scale, and normal pH is also considered alkaline. Alkaline is a positive state for the body to be in, however, it is not healthy to be too alkaline because this has the potential of slowing down the organ systems which can be dangerous to the organs. On the opposite end of that, an excessively acid state in the body is also very dangerous. A highly acidic body depletes nutrients and releases energy from the food faster than the body can consume it making the body a suitable host for disease. High acid diets also cause alkaline minerals to be lost in urination. Mineral drain results in a malnourished state of health. Cancer and most other diseases can only survive in an acid environment.

A pH imbalance is specific to the inability to use carbohydrates and fats. It produces gland problems in the endocrine system in such glands as the adrenal, thyroid, and pituitary. A pH imbalance can also produce kidney and respiratory problems. The body's hormonal levels are also affected in the levels of estrogen, progesterone, and testosterone. Maintaining a healthy pH means being conscious of what is put in the body and taking the preventative measure of checking the pH periodically to monitor health.

If your client's reading is neutral, then whatever they're doing in terms of their food intake is working for their body.

Balancing the pH has everything to do with food intake, every food also has a pH level and the body takes on the particular pH level of foods eaten. Therefore, if one eats an overwhelming amount of acid foods then the body's pH will reflect that pH level and vice-versa with alkaline. Ideally a person should eat eighty percent alkaline foods and twenty percent acid foods. Which means that a plant-based eating lifestyle has proven to be best because eighty percent of the fruits and vegetables that are available to the consumer are alkaline, and about twenty percent of the other foods like grains, meats and a few vegetables are acid. The following list confirms this point.

pH Food Chart

Alkaline Foods

Apple	Apricot	Avocado	Banana
Blackberry	Blueberry	Cantaloupe	Cherry
Currant	Grapes	Grapefruit	Honeydew
Lemon	Lime	Mango	Nectarine
Orange	Papaya	Peach	Pear
Persimmon	Pineapple	Raisins	Raspberry
Strawberry	Tangerine	Watermelon	Beet
Bell pepper	Broccoli	Burdock	Cauliflower
Chives	Garlic	Eggplant	Ginger
Kale	Lentil	Lettuce	Mushroom
Okra	Onion	Parsley	Parsnip
Potato	Pumpkin	Sweet Potato	Squash
Yam	Oats	Quinoa	Wild rice
Almonds	Flax seeds	Poppy seeds	
Pumpkin seeds		Sunflower seeds	
Sesame seeds		Brussels sprouts	
Collard greens		Mustard greens	
Sea vegetables		Turnip greens	

Acid Foods

Cranberry	Dates	Fig	Guava
Plum	Pomegranate	Prune	Tomato
Carrots	Spinach	Chickpea	Green pea
Kidney beans	Lima beans	Navy beans	Peanut
Pinto beans	Snow pea	Soy beans	String beans
Tofu	White beans	Amaranth	Barley
Brown rice	Buckwheat	Corn	Brazil nut
Hazelnut	Pecan	Pine nuts	Pistachio
Walnut	Wheat	Rye	Spelt

As you can see in the list most fruits and vegetables are alkaline and most grains and beans are acid as well as all meats and processed foods. To keep the body at a normal pH, the majority of any meal should be alkaline. However, if the body is already alkaline, then you would suggest to your client to take a higher amount of acid food to assist with bringing the pH into the normal range. If a client is a meat eater, they are not going to be overly alkaline. Meat eaters usually have pH test results that are either normal or acid based on the amount of flesh they consume.

Testing the pH
The acid and alkaline balance of the body is measured numerically in pH.

$$1\text{-}6.3 = \text{Acid}$$
$$6.4 \textit{(ideal pH)} \text{-}7 = \text{Neutral}$$
$$7\text{-}14 = \text{Alkaline}$$

An accurate reading of the body's pH is done by testing both the saliva and the urine. Alkaline is a unit of measurement on the high end of the pH scale at a measurement of 7.0 and above, pH ranges between 6.4 and 7.0 is considered normal, and a 6.4 reading is an ideal pH which shows complete balance of alkaline and acid. Also, note that a normal range of 6.4 to 7.0 is also considered alkaline. The acid range measures at 6.3 and below. Testing is done with pH paper that you can get at most drugstores. I recommend the 5.5 to 8.0 pH testing scale that is used in the Natural Health and Wellness Consultant Certification Naturopath classes taught at A Life Of Peace Wellness Education Institute.

Name brands are not important, there are a few producers of pH paper who use this scale.

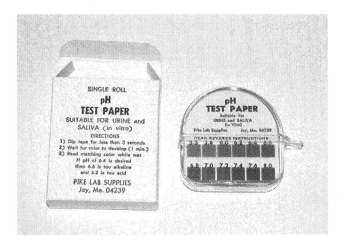

Biochemical testing of the urine and saliva reveal various indicators about the functioning of the body.

Prepare for pH testing with the following materials:
pH paper
Protective gloves
Paper towels
Urine specimen cup 4oz.
Trash can with liner or small biohazard bag

Step 1: Put on your protective gloves and lay out your paper towels for easy access.

Step 2: Tear off about an inch of the pH paper.

Step 3: Have the client to put the tip of the paper in their mouth and wet it with their saliva and take it out.

Step 4: Have your client give a small urine sample, about a third of the cup, in a clear or white plastic cup.

Step 5: Tear off another inch of the pH paper and wet the tip with urine. Withdraw it and read it immediately and record the number.

Step 6: Calculate the average pH.

The formula to compute the body's average pH includes the information obtained from both the saliva and urine.

$$\text{Urine} = U$$
$$\text{Saliva} = S$$

$$\frac{U+2S}{3} = \text{AVERAGE pH}$$

Example

Urine 7.2   Saliva 5.0

$$\frac{7.2 + 2(5.0)}{3} \qquad \frac{7.2 + 10}{3} \qquad \frac{17.2}{3} = 5.7$$

Let's say for instance the result of the urine test is 7.2 and the result of the saliva test is 5.0. The formula is the urine pH which was 7.2 plus two times the saliva pH divided by 3. 7.2 plus 2 times 5.0 equals 7.2 + 10 which equals 17.2. Next divide the top of the equation by three and the average pH is 5.7 which according to the pH chart, anything that is 6.3 or less is considered acid.

Once you determine the overall body pH, you can then help the client normalize their pH by recommending pH specific foods. It takes about seven days to alter the body's pH, however it could take longer depending on the range of pH imbalance from the neutral zone. The further away from neutral the pH is the longer the food therapy may need to be extended.

Alkaline Water and the pH

Alkaline water has become very popular in detoxing, but it is for who it's for. Meaning, if your client is in a healthy state or in a mild state of disease progress and already alkaline, they don't need to drink alkaline water every day. A client who is already a vegan or vegetarian and going through a seasonal detox, alkaline water is not recommended. Some mineral waters are naturally alkaline and fall within the neutral range, also most health-conscious individuals take in their trusted brand which will provide them the needed alkalinity. Alkaline water is like a natural medicine for those in a chronic, severe or fatal state of disease progression and acidic. Therefore, I don't recommend everyone generally drink alkaline water. Specifically, it is a great supplement for those people dealing with low levels of pH and/or who has a cigarette, alcohol, recreational drug, or marijuana addiction thereby mandating green foods and alkaline water as one of the primary requirements for detoxing.

Multistix 10 SG Urinalysis

For the Detox Therapist, the urinalysis is intended to assist in identifying and confirming stress in the kidney (urinary system), immune system, metabolism, digestive and detoxification functions. The strips also measure physical characteristics, including pH and other biochemical concentrations. With a small sample of urine this test reads the body's glucose, bilirubin, ketones, specific gravity, blood content in the urine, abnormal protein presence, urobilinogen, nitrates and leukocytes. This vital information provides the ability to know what imbalances are present. It is also a guide for the actions needed to develop an effective detox program for the client.

Prepare for the urine analysis with the following:
4oz. Container or specimen cup
Protective gloves
Paper towel
Analysis Results Form and pen
Fresh urine sample
Trash can with liner or small biohazard bag

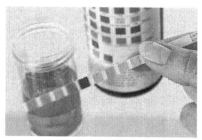

Have client void urine filling ¾ of the specimen container. Test urine immediately or within 2 hours of collection. If unable to test within the recommended time frame, refrigerate the specimen and allow it to return to room temperature before testing.

Step 1: Gather all necessary materials.

Step 2: Put on all the protective gear.

Step 3: Note color, odor and clarity.

Step 4: With gloved hands remove one strip from container taking care not to touch the testing pads on the strip and close container immediately to avoid over exposure of remaining strips.

Step 5: With a paper towel underneath the specimen cup dip the entire test strip in the urine, making sure urine covers all the test pads on the strip.

Step 6: Upon removing the strip from the urine, lightly dab it on the paper towel to tap away excess urine.

Step 7: Urine analysis is a timed test, and should be completed according to the reading times listed on the bottle key code.

Begin timing at 30 seconds and note the first test reading (glucose) and continue to monitor the time per test while recording results.

Record the results in an organized manner on your notepad or create a form for easy fast recording.

Color: Straw/Amber   Colorless   Orange   Milky
        Yellow   Brown   Red   Green
        Black
        Indication:

Clarity: Clear   Smokey Turbidity   Mucous
        Indication:

Odor: Low   Sweet   Ammonia   Offensive
        Indication:

	Positive	Negative
Glucose		
Bilirubin		
Ketones		
Specific Gravity		
Blood Hemolyzed		
Non-Hemolyzed		
Protein		
Urobilinogen		
Nitrite		
Leukocytes		

Multistix 10 SG Urine Analysis Interpretations

Color

Straw to amber - normal
Colorless - alcohol ingestion, kidney stress, pancreas stress
Orange - liver stress, dehydration, infection
Milky - bacterial infection
Brown - liver stress
Yellow - dehydration
Red - infection, presence of blood
Black - liver stress, kidney stress, metabolism stress

Transparency
Clear - normal
Low Turbidity (unclear w/ small debris)
low infection, poor diet
High Turbidity (unclear w/ heavy debris)
strong infection

Odor
Low - normal
Sweet – pancreas stress, liver stress, presence of excess sugars
Ammonia - bacterial growth, loss of alkaline buffers
Offensive - possible inflammation, toxicity

Glucose (measures the sugar content of the urine)
Positive - check for diabetic tendencies, indicates glucose spill in urine, kidney stress

Bilirubin (product of red blood cell breakdown and is normally eliminated in the bile)
Positive - heart stress, liver stress, inflammation, red blood cells weak due to poor absorption

Ketone (fats turn to sugar)
Positive - alcohol use, poor carbohydrates use, high protein diet, dehydration, pancreas stress, digestive stress, kidney stress - kidneys can't eliminate ketones efficiently switches to using fats for energy

Specific Gravity (weight of urine caused by minerals content) 1.015 Healthy specific Gravity
Above 1.015 - high intake of water, kidney stress, inefficient mineral absorption
Below 1.015 – dehydration, pancreas stress, kidney stress, overactive adrenal glands (i.e. stress) too much salt

Blood
Hemolyzed (split red blood cells)
liver stress

Non-hemolyzed (unsplit red blood cells)
kidney stress, inflammation, blood pressure stress, infection

Urine pH (speed of digestion)
6.5 to 7.0 normal urine pH
7.0 to 8.0 alkaline - infection from urea - slow digestion
5.0 to 6.0 acid - digestion and absorption stress, kidney stress, heart stress, undigested food

Protein (a small amount is normal; however excessive amounts indicate imbalances)
Positive – dehydration, kidney stress or inflammation, heart stress causing hypertension

Urobilinogen (intestinal bacteria acting on bile from the liver) 0.2 – 1 mg/dL - normal secretion
2 – 8mg/dL - blood cells dying due to toxicity or

infection, liver losing ability to make digestive enzymes, liver inflammation and blockage, spleen dysfunction

Nitrites (in regular blood pressure, dilates veins and arteries, helps muscle spasms)
Positive - bacterial proliferation in urinary tract

Leukocytes (white blood cells filtered from the body after being killed from fighting off infection)
Positive – infection, white blood cells are deficient due to inadequate diet

The physical assessment however, is only a small part of the detox assessment. It is also vital to know what is going on in the client's life and the health of their emotional, mental and spiritual well-being. The following questions can be used as a guide to peer into the depths of the soul.

Detox Consultation Questionnaire
Please read each statement carefully and select the honest answer.

STATEMENTS
    I have experienced recent hair loss.
    I have occasional or frequent headaches.
    I have an acne problem.
    I have excessive mucus build up in the lungs.
    I smoke.

I have sudden cough flare ups.
I am fatigued in some areas of my body.
I have a consistent exercise regimen.
I have normal sexual function.
I have taken over the counter medications in the past year.
I sleep well, and get 6 – 8 hours of sleep a night.
I drink soda.
I eat candy.
I eat meat.
I use salt in my food.
I eat processed foods.
I eat out at restaurants.
I drink alcohol.
I am overweight.
I am obese.
I have back pain.
I suffer from depression.
I drink at least 8 glasses of water every day.
If I eat 3 times a day, I have 3 bowels movements the same day.

All these statements reveal a health habit or issue that may contribute to an unhealthy lifestyle. Use each answer to consult with your client on recommended changes in lifestyle that will benefit their detox and long term health goals.

Chapter 6 Types of Detox

Oxygen is the body's primary cell detoxifier. It fuels all body systems; oxygen eliminates toxins and wastes and moderates the chemical reactions in the body. To begin a system of detoxification the first thing a client must do is implement a system of adding more oxygen to the cells of the body. Water would be primary in conjunction with cleansing the blood cells.

Start by eliminating known toxins in your client's lifestyle with the use of air and water filters in the home, buy or grow organic foods, use natural products for cleaning the body and home and develop a consistent detox schedule. Detoxing protects the body from disease by resting the organs through fasting or giving the body a break from processed foods which are part of the majority of people's diets.

There are a few different types of detox programs that you can take your client through, depending on the results of your assessment.

Nutritional Detox

Food vitality will be most important in your client's healing and health maintenance process. Biologically the body needs essential minerals and nutrients for full operation of the metabolic and digestive systems. Electrically a healthy diet raises the vibrational frequencies of the body's organs, tissues and cells which boost the immune and nervous systems. Chemically in conjunction with holistic thought patterns, medicinal food supplies the body with oxygen, nutrients and amino acids for building proteins which are necessary for all cellular functions, emotional health and psychological wellbeing.

In Naturopathy, the first line of recommendation to a client for the healing process involves the eating lifestyle. This will also be the case for Detox Therapists. If the nutrition component of health can be worked on with consistency, the client has a good chance of being successful in their desired health change.

The emphasis on nutrition in the detox process can never be understated. The holistic detox process is designed help bring the body, thoughts and actions back into balance with the natural rhythms of nature. Humans were designed to live in harmony with the earth and all things in it. Therefore, alignment with the life sustaining nutrient supply in the form of real food in vital. 70% of disease states in the body are food related disease. Subtle changes in the eating lifestyle of a person can rectify imbalances, however, the high percentage says there is something wrong with the mentality of people concerning food. The food industry is providing junk food and people have now become accustomed to taking what they are given for the sake of convenience. Unhealthy food must be unacceptable for all families; however, it will take a mass quantity of people to work to stop the cycle of eating and getting sick from what is consumed.

People are often in denial about their eating lifestyles, most times due to ignorance and other times due to their food addictions which have a greater control over their lives than their will to live. As a Detox Therapist, you can provide the education that is needed to enlighten clients on the balance and necessity of a healthy eating lifestyle. Each detox program that you create should include a nutrition plan specifically designed for the individual client as every person is unique.

The nutritional detox focuses on what to eat and designs an eating lifestyle that is most supportive for the client's health. How do you find out what best supports your client's health? You talk about how they live. Do they have time to prepare meals at home? Do they work extended hours every day? Do they have a lot of responsibilities when they come home such as taking care of the children, cleaning the house, etc? Do they work overnight? The client's lifestyle determines what kind of nutritional detox you put them on. Although eating plant-based meals is best for human consumption, some people do eat meat and have no intention of going strictly plant-based. Other questions to consider when planning and supporting your client are, how many times a week do they eat outside the home? Is the majority of their food consumption cooked? If so, a multivitamin may be in order for adequate nutritional needs.

Many people find it more expensive to prepare food at home than to pick up a quick meal from the local restaurant. For example, many restaurants serve value meals as a draw for consumers to eat cheap and fast. Therefore, you may also find yourself teaching clients how to choose healthy food on the run which is a very helpful component of detoxing.

Clearing the Digestive System

A clear digestive system is key to successful detoxing. A very simple way to get your client started on the road to detoxing is this natural food formula for a morning drink. There are many versions of the Natural Food Detox Formula which has at its foundation nutritional ingredients that soothe, purge, build and heal all at the same time. This formula is very mild but very effective for cleansing the stomach, small intestine and colon. It also revitalizes the immune, circulatory and excretory systems with a simple combination of foods that are widely available. This formula can be taken at the beginning and throughout the detoxification process. The client should prepare and drink this formula by the cup throughout the day.

It is recommended to divide the intake of the Natural Food Detox Formula into either four or two servings. Drink a cup in the morning, two cups in the afternoon and one cup in the evening or if the client will be on the run for the day, drink two cups before they leave and then two cups when they return home. The Natural Detox Formula gives the whole digestive system a very nice mild cleanse. It is not one of those purges that will have the client going to the bathroom uncontrollably.

The Natural Food Detox Formula helps the liver, kidneys and lungs to clear more efficiently, it purifies the blood, hydrates the body and raises the body's pH to an alkaline level. The blended formula includes water for hydration, the lemon for alkalinity, the garlic for bacteria and blood cleansing, cayenne for circulation maple syrup for nutrition and olive oil for purging the detox organs. It is an excellent all-natural cleanse.

Natural Food Detox Formula
4 cups of spring water *(provides nutrients, dilute toxins and flushes toxins)*
Juice of 1 fresh squeezed lemon *(contains water soluble vitamins)*
1-2 cloves of garlic *(boosts the immune system and cleanses infections)*
1-2 shakes of cayenne pepper *(enhances the circulatory system)*

Agave nectar or maple syrup to taste *(additional nutrients) (optional)*
¼ - ½ cup of organic extra virgin cold pressed olive oil *(stimulates flushing of the colon, liver and gall bladder)*

Live Foods: The Detox Meal
In addition to the Natural Food Detox Formula, as a focus on nutrition the client should eat as much live food as possible. Live foods provide all the vital nutrients that are needed to sustain health. When food is cooked the constant heat changes the molecular structure. Temperatures above 110° cause enzyme and nutrient destruction which makes the food become nutritionally substandard. This malnutrition makes the digestion process more difficult and often incomplete. For example, studies show that more than half the vitamin content can be destroyed in the cooking process. Broccoli has a vitamin C nutritional rating of 118 in its live state, when cooked the nutritional rating drops to 74. Live turnips have a vitamin C nutritional rating of 136 and when cooked that rating drops to 60. Live foods also have an ample supply of water that adds to natural hydration. Live foods are high in fiber and anti-oxidants. As a Detox Therapist, it is suggested that you either self-train or take classes in preparing live foods, vegan and vegetarian meals.

There is still quite a bit of education to be done surrounding live or raw foods. Although it is widely agreed that live foods have higher components of nutrients than cooked foods and live food options are more available, there is still a long way to go. Although most fruits and vegetables can be eaten in their natural state, people cook vegetation out of habit because meat must be cooked in order for it to be safe for human consumption. Therefore, the custom of steaming, roasting, frying, baking and boiling vegetation has persisted in every society of the world. Most clients in need of a detox for their health will be those who eat a majority of cooked foods and very little if any live fruits and vegetation in its natural state.

Here's the exception to the above when it comes to preparing a detox program for those who choose to consume the majority of their foods cooked. If they've never eaten live food, I make it simple for them because I want my clients to be successful:

Add a salad before everything you eat.

Beginning with a salad before eating the main meal will help the client with greater nutrient absorption, hydration, enzyme supply and digestive system function. I also teach them how to make a variety of salads to reintroduce them to the flavors of fresh foods. Even if they are eating out during their detox, most restaurants have salads on the menu that can be ordered before every meal. There are even fast food restaurants that now offer salads.

The most effective way to maximize the results of a detox program is to only consume live foods and a nonfat diet throughout the length of the program. Clients that are willing to commit to this eating lifestyle, even for a short period of time will see tremendous results in their energy, skin, weight, and more.

"Real food needs no label" is a popular adage that should be an anthem for those who would like to maintain their health. The more we consume foods in their natural state the higher our rate of absorption and the more fuel we give the body to function and regenerate at its optimal level.

Live foods are very easy to eat and prepare and the variety is endless. There are only about seven popular varieties of meats, however, the selection of fruits and vegetables far outnumber that ten times over. To take the time to prepare healthy meals has more than a few benefits. One, it allows the person to select foods that are appealing to them on a sensory level, to see and touch with the anticipation of tasting raises the energetic relationship between the person and their food. This increase in energy nurtures the digestive cellular functions. Two, to know what ingredients are in the dishes that one consumes is empowering confirmation that a person is feeding their body correctly. Three, personal food preparation is a good way to de-stress and enjoy a moment of self-care.

The varieties of live food dishes include protein rich patés, soups, porridges, salads, sandwiches, vegetable mixes, soaked grains, vegetables wraps, sea vegetable entrees, puddings, pies, cakes, and more. It is advised that as a Detox Therapist, you provide menus and food preparation classes to your clients. A sample menu will be provided in the Meal Preparation part of this chapter.

Juicing and Smoothies
A nutritional detox may also include liquid foods for fast nutritional absorption and to give the digestive tract an adequate chance to purge effectively. Juicing as a detox regimen is relative to what we term nutritional fasting. This is where a client will take in a liquid diet for a certain number of days, 1-3 days for beginners and increased days for those who make nutritional fasting a part of their regular detox lifestyle. Juice is a highly concentrated form of nutrition and dilution is recommended for all juices. High concentrations of nutrients can stress the organs more, especially the kidneys if not consumed properly.

Juice can be the initial cleanse itself. Detox juices includes all green vegetables and fruits. Green juice is the number one detox juice formula. During detox, the majority of the juice content should be vegetable based and it is wise to limit the mixing of fruits and vegetables because they have different levels of sugar components that could affect the rate of detoxing. Juice should always be made fresh with a blender or juicer and consumed immediately.

An important aspect of juicing to remember is that juicing is highly concentrated, for example if you are going to eat a serving of carrots, how many carrots would you normally eat? Most would eat one or two carrots, however, if you juice carrots for a carrot juice, usually six to ten carrots are used. This illustrates the high concentration of nutrients that is consumed in juicing. The solution to not creating organ stress with a nutritional juice fast during detoxification is to teach the client how to properly consume their juices. The naturopathic rule is half and half. A serving of juice is 8 ounces, therefore the proper combination should be 4 ounces of juice with 4 ounces of water.

If the client continuously drinks highly concentrated juices they will stress out the kidneys. The kidneys have to filter that excessive amount of minerals and vitamins, as this excess is not normal for the body. It is vital to avoid any unnecessary stress on the body during a detox program.

The second component that is vital to remember in a juice detox is the importance of vegetable juices as the primary source of nutrition. Green vegetables are filled with chlorophyll which supplies the blood with a high component of oxygen needed for the red blood cells. Vegetable juices provide potassium and natural sodium that helps the cells balance its fluid intake to maintain healthy cardiovascular function. Vegetation provides the body with the energy to maintain lightness for mobility, energy for longevity and amino acids for muscles and the body's tissues. Fruit juice on the other hand have a high level of natural sugar liquor, which binds to toxicity in the body. Natural sugar liquors cause the toxicity to be removed from the body at a very rapid rate, therefore if the client is not experienced in the detoxification process they may have the adverse effect of feeling worse before they feel the energizing effects of the detox process. Their body will go through a rapid detox that draws on the energy of the body.

If the client is experienced with the detoxification process then they can have fruit juices, if they are not experienced they only get vegetables juices. Detox juice combinations should be based on the client's nutritional needs. If a client's eating lifestyle is the standard American diet, an emphasis should be put on whole nutrition in multivitamin juice formulas.

Cool Green Drink
5 leaves of kale, 1 cup of spinach, 1 cucumber, 1 cup of spring water

Juice vegetables through the juicer, combine with water and serve. Serves 2.

Nutrients: beta carotene, calcium, iron, copper, manganese, folic acid, magnesium, chlorophyll, silica, potassium, vitamins A, B1, B2, B6, C, E and K.

Body Nourishment: Regulates the body's pH, high in antioxidants, nourishes the eyesight, respiratory system and the connective tissue, builds muscles, ligaments, tendons, cartilage and bone, protects against macular degeneration, cataracts, cancer, skin, swelling and burns.

Goddess Healing Potion
1 oz. of wild blue green algae juice, 2 oz. ginger juice fresh squeezed, 5 oz. natural water, 1 tsp. agave nectar

Stir in a 12oz. glass and enjoy the rich tantalizing burst of energy! Serves 1.

Nutrients: Vitamin B-12, B complex, chlorophyll, protein, iron, beta-carotene, calcium, vitamins C and A, folic acid, biotin, niacin

Body Nourishment: Alleviates congestion, aids in digestion, use for vitamin and mineral deficiencies, heavy metal poisoning, purifies the blood, stops inflammation, rejuvenates cells, anemia, obesity, dermatitis, yeast over growth, depression, enhances memory, supports the hypothalamus, the pineal and pituitary glands, contains phycocyanin which are pigments that prevent cancer clusters.

Smoothie Nutritional Detox works very similar to juicing; however it is a bit more filling as liquid nutrition. All standards for juicing apply to smoothies as well. Green vegetables are emphasized and the nutritional value of smoothies always taken into consideration People have a perception that a smoothie is sweet fruits and juices, however all detox smoothies should have a protein base with fruit added as a flavor enhancer.

Smoothies are a blend of vegetables and/or fruits that provide nutrition and fiber as a liquid meal. Most people tend to drink a very large smoothie, however a serving size on any smoothie is 12 ounces. Smoothies can be a meal replacement at any time of the day during detoxification. Provide different types of smoothie recipes for your client based on their nutritional needs and always include green smoothies.

Food combining can also be a consideration when blending smoothies. Melon smoothies should just include melon. This is the only fruit that is not recommended to be mixed with any other fruits. For example, a cantaloupe smoothie would just include cantaloupe, water, a little sweetener and ice, which is optional.

The following list of acid, sub-acid and sweet fruits is a guide to the most popular fruits that are used in smoothies that go well together based on their biochemistry. Food combining is important for the way the body naturally processes food density.

Acid	Sub-acid	Sweet
strawberries	peaches	bananas
cherries	apples	papaya
oranges	grapes	dates
pineapple	mango	kiwi

Some examples of good food combing for smoothies include:
strawberry/mango/pineapple
cherry/ apple
kiwi/ pineapple/ mango
kiwi/ orange/ apple
grapes/ mango/ cherry
mango/ orange
peaches/ banana/ dates
mango/ banana/ dates
papaya/ banana/ dates
papaya/ mango/ dates

Green vegetable smoothies are usually combined with fruits, however, ideally vegetables and fruit should be eaten separately. Some of the most popular green smoothie combinations include:
Spinach/ parsley/ alfalfa
Wheatgrass/ mint/ celery
Kale/ beet greens/spinach

lettuce/ celery/ beet greens
spinach/ aloe/ wheatgrass
lettuce/ parsley/ spinach
spinach/ celery
kale/ cucumber/ beet greens
collard/ lettuce/ cucumber
wheatgrass/ mint/ cucumber

Using water or nut milk base for vegetable smoothies makes the blending easier and adds flavor to the mix.

In liquid nutrition detox, the juice and smoothie is intended to be a liquid meal that provides the organs a rest for the regeneration process. Liquid nutrition can also be combined with nutritional solid meals during a detox regimen.

Nutritional Meals

The proven way of achieving the desired goals in detoxing is through nutrition. Detoxification always involves eating lifestyle improvements and changes that will move your client to living a healthier lifestyle. It is also recommended that in addition to taking the detoxification certification, that you also take a course to study different types of nutritional eating to be able to assist all clients and gain a greater understanding of what nutrients are important for the body and meal planning. A Detox Therapist is also a nutrition consultant because you will be working with nutrition planning for each of your clients. It would also be good if your own eating lifestyle reflects healthy eating, that way you can assist your clients based on experience. Having a variety of nutritional recipe books that you are familiar with is another great asset for formulating meal plans.

If you have a client that has a busy lifestyle it would be good to know the healthy selections at the popular restaurants and cafes to help the client choose food that supports their detox program. If your client is inclined and dedicated to preparing their own meals, have different recipes available for their use. Always follow up with your client on their meal planning and get feedback from your clients on their successes and challenges.

Meals should also be planned according to time. Upon waking consume a protein rich meal, the heaviest meal of the day should be lunch which includes a generous amount of vegetables, concentrated protein, and grains, nuts or seeds, every day during the detox program. Evening meals before 8:00pm should be light vegetation. A heavy meal at night slows the regenerative process that the body has to go through each night. When the body has to process a heavy meal in the stomach it will prioritize the need of the body, which is regenerating the cells. Therefore, night eaters find themselves waking up in the middle of the night uncomfortably bloated, or feeling sluggish in the morning and less hungry because the undigested food is still present in the stomach.

A weekly check in with your client when they choose meal planning will help support their consistency and change process. After they have gone through a week, Monday to Friday, schedule for them to check in with you on Saturday for therapy and to look at what worked that week and what didn't work to make the second week even more successful. The check in also allows them the chance to let you know what they liked or didn't like about the menu, which is very important towards success too.

Sample Menu of Recipes
Monday
    Power Boost Almond
    Smoothies are quick and easy for the morning rush.
    Warm Spinach Salad
    Plantain Salad
    New intros to the family are with foods they are familiar with.

Tuesday
    Mango Munch
    The Best Veggie Sandwich in the World
    Lunches should be hearty and the heaviest meals of the day.
    Mixed Greens Delight

Wednesday
    Avocado Heaven
    Kale Salad with Walnut Pate
    Fresh Greens Salad

Thursday
- Blueberry Smoothie
- Carrot Tuna Sandwich
- Hot Greens

Friday
- Strawberry Blessings
- Vegan Pizza
- Chocolate Ball Surprise
- *Vegan desserts are always a winner even with the meat eaters.*

Sample Recipe Layout

Monday

Power Boost Almond

1 cup of almonds (soaked overnight)

1 organic banana (frozen for thicker smoothie)

¼ cup of organic oats

1 cup organic almond milk

1 tbs. flaxseed oil

1 tbs. organic agave nectar

Combine all ingredients and blend well. Pour and enjoy. This is an excellent source of morning protein to get the brain going for the day.

Warm Spinach Salad

½ lb of organic baby spinach

1 organic avocado

½ cup organic cherry tomatoes cut in halves

½ Tbsp. of organic virgin olive oil

½ tsp of organic flaxseed oil

1 hand full of raw oats
1 Tbsp. of liquid aminos

Mix all ingredients in a large bowl. Mix well with your loving hands well and serve. Serves 2

Plantain Salad
1 ripe plantain
½ stalk of green onion
½ tbs. liquid aminos
½ tsp. curry powder
½ tsp. turmeric
¼ cup soaked almonds

Peel and slice very ripe plantain. Cut into coins. Chop green onions. Mix all ingredients, let chill for 30 minutes and serve. Serves 2

Tuesday

Mango Munch
1 large organic mango sliced off seed
1 cup of pineapple cubed
¼ cup of organic oats
1 cup rice milk or liquid of choice
1tbs. flaxseed oil
1 tbs. organic agave nectar

Combine all ingredients and blend well. Pour and enjoy.

The Best Veggie Sandwich in the World
2 slices sprouted bread
½ organic cucumber
1 organic tomato
2 whole leaves of organic green leaf or romaine lettuce
alfalfa sprouts
1 avocado
¼ tsp. garlic powder
¼ juice of a lemon

Dress your bread if desired. Lay on the lettuce, tomato, cucumber, alfalfa sprouts. Remove avocado from shell and mash and mix in a bowl with garlic powder, lemon juice and desired seasons. Top alfalfa sprouts with avocado mix, close sandwich, cut in half and enjoy. Increase ingredients based on number of people to serve.

Mixed Greens Delight
½ napa cabbage
½ green leaf lettuce
¼ green cabbage
1 cup parsley leaves

Chop and layer greens in a salad bowl.

Green Delight Dressing
2 garlic cloves
4 green onion stalks
½ jalapeno pepper

1 small bunch cilantro
1 lime, juiced
¼ cup of water
½ tsp sea salt (or to taste)
2 tsp olive oil
½ tsp cumin powder

Top greens with dressing on each individual salad.

To enhance your menu planning skills, here are a few recipe books that are a great place to start. Also look for food preparation classes in your area.

Recommended Recipe Books
Veggie Delights: Holistic Health Recipes for Maximum Nutrition ... by K. Akua Gray
Akwaaba!: Dr. Akua's Ghanaian Vegan Cuisine by K. Akua Gray
The Joy of Living Live by Zakkah Baht Isreal
Raw: The Uncook Book by Juliano
The Joy of Not Cooking by Imar Hutchins
Afro-Vegan by Bryant Terry

A common hazardous component of the kitchen that most households have come to live with is the microwave oven. In the last twenty years, every new home built comes with a microwave oven as the standard kitchen appliances. Microwaves have a nuclear chemical component that can heat up food within seconds. Think about the natural pattern of heat, there is nothing natural on Earth that can get from 0 degrees to 600 degrees in three seconds. For this reason alone, it should give one pause in considering to use such a powerful machine to cook the foods that one takes in for nutrition. This lifestyle change of discontinuing the use of the microwave may be a very difficult adjustment for some families because of the perceived convenience.

Aluminum cookware creates a health hazard through the absorption of aluminum particles into the bloodstream through digestion. Aluminum seeps into the food during cooking and baking. Aluminum is not processed by the body, instead it becomes laden in the crevices of the body's tissue and brain which can result in heavy metal poisoning. Safer cookware includes stainless steel, glass cookware, earthen pots, cast iron and copper cookware. Non-stick cookware can be just as hazardous when the non-stick coating begins to peel and slough off into the food while cooking.

Detox for Weight Loss

Nutritional Detox is also commonly used for clients to begin the weight loss process and assist with making permanent changes in their lifestyle when they are overweight or obese. Increasing the metabolism rate is important for the client to achieve permanent weight loss. The metabolism rate measures how many calories a person burns when they are in a resting position. The metabolism rate increases when the body gets moving consistently and the weight comes off when the person eats nutritionally within proportion.

Calculate Metabolism Rate

1) Take weight in pounds and divide by 2.2 to get weight in kilograms (kg).
2) Take height in inches multiply by 2.54 to get height in centimeters (cm).
3) For females: (kg weight x 9.99) + (cm height x 6.25) - (age x 4.92) – 161.
4) For males: (weight x 9.99) + (height x 6.25) - (age x 4.92) + 5.
5) Your total will give you the daily caloric count.

The intent of weight loss is to accelerate the rate that calories are used. For example: if the total is 1,345, then to raise the metabolism rate the person should create meals with foods according to their rating on the glycemic index that totals up to their calculated caloric count. Portions, water consumption and a detox movement regimen will also stimulate the metabolism.

The following foods have the lowest caloric ratings on the glycemic index (GI), and can recommended during a detox program. All have a rating of 51 or less and can include the serving size.

Food Type	GI	Serving
Vegetables		
Broccoli	15	1 cup
Cauliflower	20	1 cup
Celery	25	1 stalk
Green peas	48	½ cup
Carrots	47	1 large
Lettuce	15	2 cups
Kale	15	2 cups
Collard greens	15	2 cups
Mustard greens	15	2 cups
Peppers	15	2 cups
Seaweed	15	2 cups
Yam	37	1 cup
Fruits		
Apple	38	1 cup
Avocado	50	1 oz.
Banana	51	1 medium
Cherries	22	1 cup
Grapefruit	25	1 cup
Grapes	46	½ cup
Orange	42	½ cup
Peach	42	½ cup
Pear	38	½ cup
Prunes	29	1 cup
Grains		
Quinoa	50	½ cup

Wheat tortilla	30	1 small
Bulgur wheat	48	½ cup
Spaghetti	37	½ cup
Fettuccini	40	½ cup

Beans/Legumes/Nuts

Blackeye peas	42	½ cup
Black beans	30	½ cup
Chickpeas	28	1 cup
Navy beans	38	½ cup
Kidney beans	27	1 cup
Lima beans	32	1 cup
Lentils	29	1 cup
Soy beans	18	1 cup
Cashews	22	1 oz.
Peanuts	14	1 oz.

Beverages

Apple juice	40	4 oz.
Grapefruit juice	48	4 oz.
Orange juice	50	4 oz.

Snack Foods

Nonfat yogurt	14	1 cup
Hummus	6	¾ cup

Concentrated Protein

Tofu	18	4 oz.
Fish	30	2 oz.
Chicken	46	2 oz.

How do you know you are eating within proportion? A simple way to know is to slightly cup both hands and put them together to form a wide bowl with your hands. The proper amount of food at any meal should fit into your hands. If a person is eating more than that, they're overeating. Most restaurants serve twice as much as what is required for the average person. I recommend to my clients to prepare a proportioned plate of their meal before they start eating and immediately put the remainder of the meal into a take away container to have at their next meal.

Metabolically nutritious meals include eating a large amount of vegetables and carbohydrates preferably in live food form. Eating salads, fresh fruit and vegetable snacks, whole grains such as quinoa are ideal for raising the metabolism. Also, the proper amount of exercise for most people is anywhere from 3 to 5 times a week for 30 minutes to 45 minutes a day. Exercises that increase the heart rate such as aerobics, cycling or just a sweat producing walk every day will increase the metabolism rate. These changes must be done with consistency or the client will find themselves getting stuck on plateaus or gaining the weight back. Therefore, I recommend clients get a personal trainer, join a gym, attend a boot camp or get an exercise partner that will keep them motivated.

Detoxing to lose weight comes with a commitment and ideally a safe weight loss goal would be 1 – 3 pounds per week. If the client has a desire to lose 40 pounds, then the detox regimen would be scheduled for three months to help ensure consistency and periodic checks on the physical, mental, emotional and spiritual progress of the client.

The Sugar Problem is another factor in some client's ability to achieve weight loss. The food industry has incorporated sugar into most of the commercialized, processed, and packaged foods. A high intake of sugar can cause various problems for the body outside of obesity. Sugar is the number one cause of tooth decay. An excessive amount of sugar can also create yeast overgrowth, (commonly candida), which causes fungal infections, vaginal infections, urinary tract infections, rectal itching, or vaginal itching, eczema, psoriasis, hives, seasonal allergies, itchy ears, chronic fatigue, arthritis, bloating, constipation, diarrhea, poor memory, poor concentration, brain fog, mood swings, anxiety and sugar cravings. Sugar cravings which lead to frequent excessive intake of sugar is cited as a cause in nutritional deficiencies due to filling the body with empty calories. Sugar is also a factor in those with diabetes diagnosis and should be limited or eliminated by those who suffer from hyperglycemia. Sugar also has paralytic effects on the immune system which weakens the it's ability to function at its full capacity. For women, eating excessive amounts of sugar can contribute to menstrual irregularity and for children over consumption can cause hyperactivity. There are many consequences for the body when processed sugar is a primary part of any eating lifestyle.

A sugar detox is a viable way to break sugar addiction. The first aspect of a client's recovery is to take sugar consumption seriously. Most people with sugar addictions developed them in childhood and it becomes standard operating procedure to eat sweet treats, desserts, chewing gum, candy for meals, and drinking sweetened beverages. It becomes a way of life and it is always available by the food industry. A good way to have clients come to the realization of how much sugar they consume is to keep a daily journal of sweet products they ingest and also note when they have sugar cravings, even if they do not fulfill them. This analysis usually reveals the degree of severity of the sugar addiction.

Once it is established that the client would also like to include a sugar detox component to their care plan, the first recommendation should be to **increase their vegetable, whole grain and plant based proteins intake**. This must come with a commitment to **omit sugar from all food preparation** and learn to taste the natural flavors of food. **Drinking the appropriate amount of water** curbs sugar cravings. Beating the sugar addiction is intensified with a thorough look at the level of glucose in the blood, so it is recommended for the client to **have a diabetes screening**. Lastly, developing an exercise regimen that helps the body to burn fat is useful in reducing cravings.

Sometimes it takes years for people to kick their sugar addiction and sometimes a person can eliminate the addiction very quickly. It's different for everybody.

Herbal and Supplement Detox

Next to nutrition, herbs are the second most preferred method of detoxing. As the original drug (dried plant) herbals are an excellent addition to most detox plans. The results of your client's assessment will facilitate the herbal recommendations for their detox program. There are several categories of herbals for the needs of the client. It is also necessary to carefully assess what pharmaceuticals or over the counter medications your client is taking to avoid mixing herbs and chemical medications that may cause an adverse reaction. Although herbal remedies are quite useful in detoxing, your knowledge of proper use of these natural plant-based medications is of the utmost importance. If you have not taken an herbalist training course that teaches the drug and herbal interactions, nutritional foundation and biochemical reactions of herbal medicines, it would be wise to further your education prior to recommending any herbal therapies to any of your clients. Until this knowledge is gained the better choice for you in recommending herbs would be to work with proven formulas from qualified herbal companies that have laid the framework already for detoxification programs.

Detox Herbal Categories

Antibiotics kills germs, bacteria and boosts immune system functions. For example, goldenseal, chaparral, garlic, myrrh, wormwood and echinacea. When a client is having a hard time fighting infection, antibiotics in three day intervals can be recommended.

Blood Purifiers eliminate infections and remove toxins from the body through the blood and liver. For example, red clover, echinacea, dandelion, burdock and oregon grape. Bad breath, candida, liver stress, alcohol consumption, marijuana smoking and substance abuse call for blood purifiers in the detoxification process. Depending on the length of the detox program, they are taken three days of each week of detoxing.

Decongestants break up excessive amounts of mucus to clear the respiratory and digestive systems. For example, sage, hyssop, garlic, yarrow and boneset.

Diuretics increase the flow of urine to relieve water logged organs, strengthen the kidneys, and enhance weight loss. For example, uva ursi, juniper berries, parsley, yarrow and corn silk. Diuretics can relieve swelling and puffiness around the eyes.

Integumentary herbs provide regeneration to the skin. For example, peppermint, burdock, goldenseal. Use these herbs with clients with severe acne, sores and wounds.

Purging Herbs are herbal laxatives that flush out the digestive system. For example, licorice, slippery elm, cascara sagrada, senna leaf, dandelion or taking a detox herbal formula such as New Body Products CKLS (colon, kidney, liver, spleen). This is very effective, for those who only need to detox annually. CKLS is a complete organ detox in the form of a mixture of herbs. As a deep cleansing formula, it is recommended that for a first-time user, they start the cleanse on the weekend when they are not at work. Otherwise they will be making frequent runs to the toilet during this purge.

Stimulating Herbs boosts metabolism and circulation. For example, cayenne, ginger, garlic and cloves. These herbs help intensify workouts, naturally raise the metabolism and burn fat.

Toning Herbs regenerates energy in the organs and increases vitality. For example, dandelion, parsley and goldenseal. They are excellent for assisting the body in repairing itself from disease, injury and increasing mass.

Tranquilizers calm nervous tension and balances

energy. For example, comfrey, barley, valerian, kava kava, skullcap, and black cohosh. For clients who need a natural way to ease the stress of living, increase calm interactions, and reset proper sleep patterns, these herbs work with relaxing nerves and altering the biochemical functions of the brain that cause anxiety.

Herbal detox regimens can be the exclusive purging process or it can be both the purging and the toning. The selection of herbs and methods of applications will always be client specific with the most popular methods being capsules, pills, teas and tonics. Since Detox Therapists are not allowed to write prescriptions, it is advisable to inform the client to follow the label instructions of the recommended herbal formula, in accordance with the number of days in the detox program.

Consideration must also be taken when your client is taking pharmaceutical medications. In modern therapeutic herbology it is very necessary to cross reference detox herbals to avoid possible adverse effects in your client's health based on medically treated diseases.

Below is a listing of <u>NON-INTERACTIVE HERBS AND THEIR DETOX USES</u>. Also following this listing is a current list of the most common <u>INTERACTIVE HERBS AND THE PHARMACEUTICAL MEDICATIONS THEY SHOUND NOT BE USED WITH.</u>

BASIL helps the immune system with antioxidants and germ fighting qualities. It is also antimicrobial.

BLACK BERRY is a good addition to a tonic for liver regeneration.

BLESSED THISTLE destroys parasites, carries oxygen to the brain, strengthens the heart and lungs, repairs the liver, stimulates appetite, reduces pain, cleanses the blood and improves circulation.

BLUEBERRY regenerates eyesight, arteries, and veins. It is also anti-inflammatory and supplies the body with antioxidants.

BURDOCK supplies antioxidants, has antibacterial and anti-fungal properties, eliminates acne, boils, gout, arthritis and cancer cells. It is a blood purifier, diuretic and immune system booster. Use burdock for digestion especially with liver and gallbladder issues. It is also good for scalp and hair health.

BUTCHER'S BROOM relieves hemorrhoids, edema, carpal tunnel syndrome, varicose veins, and is anti-inflammatory. It is good for the urinary system, helps the circulatory system. urine flow, bladder, kidneys, and obesity.

CAROB is used for cholesterol heartburn, bacterial infection, cancer and diabetes. It is also anti-viral and anti-fungal.

CAT'S CLAW is an immune system booster, reduces the risk of heart attack, stroke, high blood pressure and cholesterol.

CHAPARRAL relieves tumors and infection.

CHICKWEED fights obesity and regulates cholesterol.

CINNAMON helps cells respond to insulin and reduces blood sugar levels.

COMFREY helps heal bone fractures, relieves stomach ulcers, congestion, and improves kidney and bowel health. It is also a blood cleanser

DAMIANA is a female energy sex stimulant that increases the libido and regenerates the reproductive organs. It also repairs the nerves and intestinal muscles.

ELDERBERRY is a detoxifying laxative, diuretic and works as an anti-inflammatory agent.

EUCALYPTUS works as an antiseptic and mucilaginous, relieves respiratory ailments, arthritis, and is a muscle relaxant.

FEVERFEW improves circulation, relieves migraine

headaches, and calms the nerves.

GOTU KOLA produces energy, eases depression, promotes longevity, improves memory, regenerates nerves and the heart tissue, lowers blood pressure, increases the sex drive, improves circulation, provides increased oxygenation, and is used to relieve asthma, dementia, eczema, pain, and kidney stress.

HOPS is used to reverse alcohol addiction, relieve insomnia, and ease pain.

HORSERADISH is used for urinary tract infection, relieves congestion and can be used as an anti-bacterial remedy.

HYSSOP is used for respiratory ailments.

KUDZU eliminates substance abuse addictions, acts as an anti-cancer agent, tones the digestive system, and is used for heart tissue regeneration.

LAVENDER eases anxiety, is used for candida, gout, lupus, headaches, insomnia, nausea, irritable bowel syndrome, and high blood pressure. It is also a good insect repellent.

MULLEIN regenerates the lungs, eases pain, breathing problems, and reduces swollen glands.

MYRRH is a powerful antiseptic, disinfectant and anti-inflammatory herb. It is also used for indigestion, ulcers, and arthritis.

NONI is used for cancer, diabetes and as an immune booster.

OATS relieve anxiety, stress, eczema, psoriasis and high cholesterol.

OLIVE LEAF is used for cancer, an anti-fungal for the skin, hair growth, and heart regeneration.

ONION assists with allergies, respiratory ailments, cancer, candida, worms and herpes.

OREGANO is used for lupus, headaches, arthritis and skin conditions.

PAU D'ARCO is a bitter herb that is high in iron, calcium, selenium, vitamins A, B-Complex and C, potassium, sodium and zinc. It is used as an antibiotic, antioxidant, anti-viral, laxative, antipyretic, diuretic, anti-malarial, and as an anti-inflammatory herb. Pau d'arco is also used in pain relief, as a blood purifier in cancer treatment including leukemia, as a blood purifier, for ulcers, diabetes, psoriasis, Hodgkin's disease, yeast infections, skin disease, sore throats, snake bites, constipation, arthritis, bed wetting, boils, acidosis, liver, gallbladder issues and the treatment of AIDS.

PEPPERMINT eases nausea, respiratory congestion, headache, irritable bowel syndrome, chills, colic and diarrhea. It also freshens bad breath.

PERIWINKLE is used for respiratory ailments, high blood pressure, diarrhea and diabetes.

PLANTAIN is used as a laxative, respiratory cleanser, blood purifier, astringent for insect bites, wounds, blisters, burns, and snake bites.

PUMPKIN relieves urinary tract infection, cholesterol, kidney and prostate stress.

ROSEMARY has ursolic acid which inhibits the breakdown of neurotransmitters critical to memory, fights free radicals, bacteria and fungus, helps to detox the liver, is a decongestant and relieves muscle cramps.

SAGE relieves night sweats, expels worms, stops bleeding wounds, cleans ulcers and sores and dries up breast milk.

SANDALWOOD is an insect repellent, eases bronchitis, insomnia and regenerates the skin.

SASSAFRAS is used as an insect repellent, for arthritis, as an antibacterial agent and for pain.

SLIPPERY ELM is used for the stomach, bowels and kidneys.

STEVIA is used for diabetes, weight loss and as a sugar substitute.

TEA TREE eliminates canker sores, lice, ulcerous tissue, poison ivy, poison oak, ringworm, athlete's foot, acne, boils, cuts, fungal infection, insect/spider bites, vaginitis and earache.

THYME reduces bouts of coughing, relieves fever, headache, liver disease, candida, itchy scalp, asthma, bronchitis and excessive mucus build up and works as an antiseptic against inflammation of the throat.

TUMERIC is used with heart disease and diabetes, relieves chronic pain, rheumatoid arthritis, reduces inflammation of the body that causes pain by inhibiting cell enzymes that contribute to inflammation.

WOOD BETONY relieves fevers, diarrhea and pain. It is also used in regenerating the blood, liver and spleen.

YARROW is used for diarrhea, fungus, the liver and pancreas.

YELLOW DOCK is high in iron, used for varicose veins, and blood ailments.

YUCCA is a natural cortisone, relieves arthritis and reduces inflammation.

Common Herbs and Interactions

Aloe – heart medications *(affects cardiac rhythm)*, diabetes medications *(induces hypoglycemia)*, diuretics *(hypokalemia, potassium loss)*

Arnica – anticoagulants: prevents blood clotting *(increases the effect)*

Astragalus - anticoagulants: *(increases the effect)*, immunosuppressant *(counteracts this type of drug)*

Bilberry - anticoagulants: *(increases the effect)*, salicylate: used in pain medications and acne medications *(increases prothrombin time)*

Brewer's Yeast – antidepressants *(increases blood pressure)*

Cascara Sagrada – heart medications *(increased effect, potassium loss)*

Cayenne – heart medications *(increases the effect)* diuretics, asthma medications *(increases absorption causing toxicity)*

Chamomile – chemotherapy *(causes interference)*,

anticoagulants *(increases the risk of bleeding)*, sedatives *(increases effect)*

Cranberry – blood thinners *(increases effect)*

Dandelion – diuretics *(increases effect)*

Dong quai – blood thinners *(increases effect)*

Echinacea – chemotherapy *(causes interference)*, immunosuppressant *(counteracts this type of drug)*

Feverfew - anticoagulants *(increases the effect)*

Fenugreek – blood thinners, hypoglycemic medications *(increases effect)*

Garlic – blood thinners, anti-inflammatory, pain medications

Ginger – chemotherapy, blood thinners

Ginkgo Biloba – anti-inflammatory, anticonvulsants *(may cause seizures in epileptics)*, blood thinners *(increases the effect)*, diabetes medications, diuretics *(may increase high blood pressure)*

Goldenseal – anti-viral medications, antibacterial medications

Green Tea – muscles relaxants, diuretics *(decreased absorption)*, anticoagulants *(interferes with drug action)*

Lemon balm – thyroid medications *(increases effect)*

Licorice – anti-inflammatory, diuretics, steroids, anticoagulants, oral contraceptives

Lobelia – nicotine alternatives *(increases effect)*

Milk Thistle – anti-inflammatory, chemotherapy, Alzheimer's medications

Psyllium – pain medications, ulcer medications, diabetes medications

Red Raspberry – pain medications, diarrhea medications

Saw Palmetto – anticoagulants *(increased risk of bleeding)*, hormone therapies *(interferes with male and female hormone therapies)*

Senna – heart medications, diuretics *(hypokalemia, potassium loss)*, estrogen therapy *(decreases hormone levels)*

St. John's Wort – heart medications, HIV medications, birth control, blood thinners

Uva Ursi – pain medications, diuretics *(increases effect)*

Valerian – sedatives, muscle relaxants *(increases effect)*

White Willow – anti-inflammatory, anti-viral, digestive system medications

Wild Yam – birth control therapies *(increases effect)*

Witch Hazel – heart medications, pain medications, decongestants, appetite suppressants

There are also a few nutritional supplements of vitamins and minerals that are beneficial for detoxing. Calcium, magnesium, and vitamin C provide nutrition to multiple functions of the body during cleansing. Calcium and magnesium used for purging and vitamin C, as a water-soluble nutrient, also assist with flushing toxins from the body.

Some additional beneficial nutritious plants include wild blue green algae, wheatgrass, spirulina and liquid chlorophyll. All of which are excellent nutritional supplements to stimulate the health of the blood and bones.

When recommending herbs for detoxing, it is a good idea to survey the lifestyle of your client to ensure you help them choose the most convenient way to take their herbs for consistency. These are referred to as methods of application. **Capsules, pills and tinctures** are good for people who are on the go and can easily work their herbs into their day at any time. Tinctures can be consumed by mouth straight from the dropper or in a glass of water or juice very quickly. **Teas and tonics** are for those who have preparation time and may be more flexible in terms of their busyness. Teas are usually single ingredient herbs, while tonics are often mixtures of herbs for purging, blood cleansing and toning. Most herbs are available in all methods of application, and if there are particular herbs that come in loose powders, they can always be encapsulated for convenience. Always discuss with your clients the best method of taking herbs that will help them be successful in their detox.

It is also good to have these herbs on hand for your clients to purchase directly from you. All wellness service businesses should have multiple streams of income and consulting and product supplying go hand in hand.

Chapter 7 Detox Therapy

So far detoxing sounds like a lot of hard work and commitment to change, however, remember the subtitle of this book "Detoxing Should Feel Good Too." The therapy component in detoxing is overlooked in most programs. Stimulating the nervous system, the endocrine system and integumentary system is not only good for the detox process, it is excellent for cellular memory when the body is going through changes. When the body experiences something pleasant and exhilarating, the cells get programmed with the desire to repeat the actions. Detox Therapy is an array of therapies that assist with commitment and comfort while detoxing. Detox Therapy involves nurturing the physical needs of the client, emotional balancing through the processes of releasing toxicity, the mental encouragement needed to ensure success and the spiritual support to make the changes for a lifetime of self-love.

Hydrotherapy Detox

Hydrotherapy is using water to assist with the detox process. Hydrotherapy can be as simple as an herbal bath, however, it can also include steam, saunas, hydro-wraps, colon therapy, whirlpool, and ion foot detox therapy. Any form of hydrotherapy that is not done with natural water should be filtered before use.

Herbal Bath therapy is used to reduce stress, relax the muscular system, nourish and soften the skin, purge impurities and saturate the circulatory system with herbs for regeneration. Use a tub full of warm to hot water. Herbs can be introduced to the body fresh, dried, loose, in a sachet or with essential oils. Bath sachets are put straight into the bath and allowed to steep 5 minutes. The body is then submerged and soaked for 15 – 30 minutes. After bath skin can be gently rubbed with terrycloth to exfoliate the skin or the body should be allowed to air dry. Herbal baths are most effective in the evening before bed when the body is preparing to activate its regeneration processes for the night. Single dried herbs are always recommended first. See the non-interactive herb listing on page 110 for what your client may need. Also remembering to use the non-interactive herb list is best in recommending blends. Herbal mixtures can include relaxation and medicinal herbs in equal parts,

Hydro-wraps can be a self-taught therapy that uses all -natural ingredients over the entire body or key areas like the back, abdomen or legs. The wraps are layers of warm to hot wet sheets or towels enveloping the body covered by dry towels or blankets wrapped tightly after natural elements of black moor mud, dead sea mud, green clay, herbs or moisturizing oils have been applied to the skin. This is a very relaxing form of rejuvenation. Once wraps are applied the client can remain wrapped with soft background music for about

15 - 30 minutes. Depending on the method of the wrap, a shower for rinsing may be necessary when finished.

A nice home personal detoxing therapy can be recommended too. Have the client to apply the mud or clay to their body and lie out in the sun with the blanket on which eliminates the need to use the hot towels. The heat from the sun helps to open the pores. The hydro-wraps also provide mineral nutrition to the body.

Whirlpools are a jet powered spa bath that is used to relax the muscular, nervous and circulatory systems and purge impurities from the skin. The standard health department regulated maximum temperature for a whirlpool to be is 102° Fahrenheit and the average length of time for hydrotherapy is 15 – 30 minutes two times a week. When using a hot tub for detox sanitation is a key factor to consider because of the number of bacteria that exist and breed in warm wet environments. There are portable whirlpool home spas available for more control over the sanitation needed for effective therapy and it eliminates the harsh chemicals that are used in sanitizing public whirlpools. In the personal whirlpool bath, the water can be natural or filtered water. Whirlpools are also good for raising the metabolism for the client who is trying to lose weight. It is not recommended to use herbs in a whirlpool, as the heat and massaging action is enough to stimulate the body to release.

Steam is a common way to detoxify the body. Sweating to purify the body is very effective in a detox program. Steam opens the pores and increases the heart rate which stimulates the integumentary and circulatory systems, which increases the blood flow, and the secretion of sweat helps to breakdown and release toxins, fat, dead cells and lymphatic fluids through the skin. The temperature of the steam room or under the steam tent should be between 90° - 120° F. Therapies are recommended for 10 – 30 minutes and can be used with aroma therapy, skin exfoliates and internal detox treatments. One example of this is the castor steam. A steam tent is used over a standard massage table for this therapy. Castor oil is applied to the limbs or the entire body. Steam is then channeled into the tent through fixated tubing to fill the tent space and starts the purging process. Depending on the client's ability to tolerate the heat, the therapy can last up to 45 minutes. After the steam is complete the skin can be brushed to remove dead skin and impurities. Clients can then wipe themselves dry or proceed directly to the shower if it is available to cleanse away any released and remaining toxic debris.

Remember, the client must hydrate by drinking natural water after any sweating therapy.

Sauna – A dry sauna or infrared sauna is a system of cleansing, detoxification and relaxation with heat to induce sweating. The temperature of the dry sauna should be between 160° - 194° F and the safe length of time to be in a dry sauna is 20 minutes – 1 hour with a five-minute break every twenty-minutes. The sauna, through a constant influx of dry heat facilitates a full body sweat. This type of thorough sweat opens the integumentary system to release toxins, fat, oil build up, and excessive fluids from the body through the pores of the skin. It should be followed by a gradual cool down process usually a bath, cool shower or an air dry.

Colon Therapy is a procedure to flush "built-up" toxins from the bowel. The treatments are given in a colon therapy office or clinic by a certified colon therapist. During the session, the client lies on a treatment table while the therapist gently inserts a small rigid tube called a speculum about $5^1/_2$ inches into the rectum. The therapist will then attach the speculum to a plastic hose connected to a colon irrigation machine. This device will slowly fill the five-foot length of the colon with warm, purified water. Herbs or enzymes are sometimes added to the water in hopes of increasing the benefits of the treatment. The water causes the muscles that line the colon to contract and expand rhythmically, forcing out the fecal matter (undigested food, water, and bacteria), gas and mucus through an evacuation tube that leads back to the machine for safe draining. While the water is in the bowel, the therapist may massage portions of the abdomen to help loosen and remove as much fecal material as possible from the pockets and folds that line the walls of the colon. Some therapists also find reflexology and special breathing and relaxation techniques useful for ridding the colon of waste. After the first infusion of water has been expelled, the procedure will be repeated until a total of 20 to 30 gallons of water have been flushed through the bowel. The client should not have any pain, but, they may feel a sensation of warmth as the cleansing proceeds.

After the session, colon therapists typically advise eating easy-to-digest, nourishing foods such as vegetable soups and broths, fruit and vegetable juices, or peppermint tea to help restore the bacterial balance in the colon. Each session lasts between 30 and 50 minutes. Some therapists advise 1 or 2 sessions in a given period of time, and others recommend 4 to 8, whereas a few therapists insist that to maintain a well-functioning colon, you need treatments every 3 to 6 months.

Ion Foot Detox is a self-contained water detoxification system that enables the body to heal itself. It uses stainless steel electrodes. The array posts deliver an electrical current through the ionizer array which causes the water, sea salt and metal combination to generate + and − ions and allows the − ions to travel through the body and attach themselves to toxins. The toxins are then neutralized and drawn out of the body back to the pores of the feet. This process raises the user's pH to a more alkaline state. During the foot bath, the cleansing process takes place as the water interacts with a compound electric current and magnetic field structure. This body cleansing process returns cells to a healthy state. The feet are immersed in warm water. The machine is set to the correct settings and ionization levels. The client relaxes for 30 minutes while the machine completes its cycle. The suggested sessions for adults are 1 to 3 initial baths per week for 1 month. Thereafter once a week, once a month or every other month depending on the client's detox program and their state of disease progression.

You may see the excreted toxins, parasites, lymphatic fat or mucous floating in the water. The water may change color from orange, brown to black due to the release of toxic substances through the 2000 pores on the sole of each foot. The color of water reveals which organs and tissues released toxins from within the body.

Black – liver, alcohol, respiratory system
Black flakes – heavy metals, blood sugar
Brown – liver, smoking, free radicals, waste products
Bubbles – digestive system, immune system, lymphatic toxins

Dark green – gall bladder, digestive system, inflammation
Oil film – fats, triglycerides
Orange brown – joints, muscles
Red patches – blood clots
White cheese – acidic wastes (uric, lactic, or fatty acids), yeast
Yellow green – kidney, bladder, reproductive system

The ionic technique of cleansing through the feet provides a purge of all vital organs, balances the body's pH, reduces inflammation, clears up skin problems, acne, eliminates sleep problems, restlessness, reduces stress, reverses wrinkles, cures headaches, eases gout symptoms, relieves arthritis pain, cures candida and yeast infections, is good for liver detoxification, purges heavy metals, increases energy, improves sexual health, and improves memory. The internal cleansing also results in faster disease healing and injury recovery.

The ion detox machine comes in many varieties and the cost can range from $160 to $2500 for the units with the massage chair included.

Touch Therapy

Touch therapy in the detoxification process helps stimulate the nervous system, releases endorphins, realign the physical body to a healthy state and promote relaxation. When someone is seeking change, it is important to be as relaxed as possible. There are five recommended forms of touch therapy that will make the detoxification process more therapeutic and inviting.

Lymphatic Drainage Therapy
Stagnation and congestion can occur in the lymphatic system, which is the body's channel in the immune system for moving impurities from the body and supplying cells with antibodies for fighting disease. There is twice as much lymphatic fluid in the body than there is blood. This detox therapy is intended to drain the lymph nodes as a form of fluid release in the lymphatic system. The lymphatic system lies just beneath the skin and does not need deep penetration to move the lymph fluids. It is a very gentle process of stretching the skin in a clockwise motion in the direction of the drainage points of the system. This technique can be self-taught or learned through formal training and is available in most major cities. If this is your clients first detox experience, this therapy is highly recommended. Apply the lymphatic drainage technique over the entire body once in the beginning of the detox and once at the end of the program.

Therapeutic Massage
This standard method of relaxation with surface and deep tissue manipulation is excellent for any detox

program. Done by licensed massage therapists, it also assists in moving stagnation and congestion from the body tissues. Therapeutic massage is recommended weekly or bi-weekly for the duration of the client's detox program.

Shiatsu
Shiatsu is a form of healing touch in which the hands, forearms, elbows, knees and sometimes feet are used to apply pressure directly to the organ meridians through energy vortex points on the body stimulating and redistributing stagnant energy for relaxation, blood flow, muscle and organ regeneration, pain relief and emotional realignment. Recommend as a weekly therapy. A Shiatsu certification course is required to administer this therapy. Shiatsu creates the synergy that the body needs to stay healthy.

Reflexology
Reflexology is therapeutic hand and foot stimulation to adjust the lymphatic, nervous and circulatory systems. Touch of the hands and feet stimulate receptors in the brain that correspond to nerve endings connected to the internal organs. Reflexology promotes relaxation, regeneration and the elimination of stagnant energy. When done properly and consistently, reflexology can increase the flow and enhance the body's ability to process oxygen and other nutrients. Sometimes circular motions of pressure are used to increase

stimulation.

Reflexology stimulation releases endorphins, enhances enzyme function, relaxes muscle tension and aligns the body systems. Reflexology can be a self-taught method of touch therapy that involves moving the fingers and knuckles along the palms and soles, tapping the hands and feet gently, kneading and rubbing the hands and feet for nerve stimulation.

Naturopathic Reiki is a gentle therapy that provides the human experience with a limitless supply of energy to stimulate regeneration in the physical body, enhance positive outcomes in the mental body, balance the emotional body and it seeks out the essence of divinity in the spiritual body. Naturopathic Reiki is a gentle technique of touch and relaxation therapy that allows the client a moment of peace in a safe environment to just let go of the outside world in order to heal and rejuvenate. This path of Reiki was developed by Dr. Akua Gray, ND, to include the health components of naturopathy that nurture the whole client, body, mind and spirit. It is one of the forms of energy healing that can cleanse the energy body, raise low level vibration and reset the energetic functions of the organ systems. Naturopathic Reiki may be utilized by lightly touching or hovering the hands over the body in specific places where energy vortexes are located. In levels one and two of Naturopathic Reiki, there is no manipulation of the physical body, however in level three master therapists are taught tapping, smoothing and massage in conjunction with working on specific states of disease progression. Naturopathic Reiki is a gentle, loving and powerful energy medicine for both the client and the therapist. It is so relaxing to the body that the flowing energy will effortlessly heal everyone in the room.

Naturopathic Reiki is a three-level certification course taught worldwide by certified Naturopathic Reiki Masters. Naturopathic Reiki students are taught mantras, hand positions, Reiki history and the protocol for personal preparations to deliver clean energy purifications. To be able to give this kind of energy medicine a therapist must do a significant amount of self-healing which is the focus of Naturopathic Reiki in the first degree teaches a path of personal healing and self-improvement. Naturopathic Reiki in the second degree teaches how to provide an energy medicine service to others, how to use the first set of Reiki symbols and mantras and healing techniques as a beginning therapist. Naturopathic Reiki in the third degree is the master teacher level. Students learn the ability to manipulate energy and use the powerful master level symbols and mantras.

Reiki in general is very popular worldwide and it comes in many different forms however Naturopathic Reiki is one of the highest forms of Reiki in the world of alternative medicine today.

Detox Movement

If the body remains motionless, it cannot thrive, therefore, adding movement to a detox program is beneficial for the overall results for the client. Walking to sweat is detox movement to make a difference. The basic detox movement is walking; however, it is walking with the intention to release. Sweat is a natural purging process of the body and temperature regulator. It strengthens and builds muscles, promotes flexibility, endurance, stamina, positive hormonal release, respiratory health and circulatory system function. Walking should be done daily.

Encourage your client to pursue various types of movement that will boost the results of the detox. For example, aerobics, swimming, dancing, skating, cycling, jogging, tai chi, martial arts, dancing and yoga are viable choices ensuring a movement component is added to benefit the client's overall health. In the detox process, movement brings the mind, body, emotions and spirit into alignment for a lifestyle of effective change. Detox movement is highly recommended for detox programs that have a long-term requirement; it is another point of focus that promotes consistency.

Metaphysics of Detox

The metaphysics of detox is a look into the spiritual side of your client to offer encouragement and therapies that can help a person learn to live with the flow of life for a greater sense of peace. Every situation in life cannot be controlled. It is vital to learn and know how to let go of emotional, mental and physical stress that makes life hard to live. Having a wisdom system, whether it's religious or formal spirituality helps keep the mind in a state of peace. Being spiritually healthy equals being peaceful in everything.

The tools that are available to everyone for balancing life begins with speaking positive words that manifest positive experiences in life. Affirmations and chants help to restructure the thought patterns. They are reminders that life can change for the better and serves as vehicles of empowerment. When a person speaks words, and those words become a reality, their strength and determination increase. Affirmations are sweet releases of pain, failure, bad relationships, and any burdens that plague the spirit. Affirmations also increases the ability to forgive and makes accepting change more permanent. Some sample affirmations taken from <u>Today: Wellness Manifestations</u> by K. Akua Gray that are helpful during detoxing include:

- ♀ *Affirm Today*: When my spirit leads me in my first mind thoughts today, I will follow. When my spirit leads me to speak words of light today, I will let them be heard. I will walk according to my purpose. When my spirit leads me to nourish my body with the goodness of the Earth today, I will choose life and enjoy. I will live today like I KNOW who I am.

- ☥ *Affirm Today*: Today I free my soul from ignorance. I am not my body. I am the infinite peace of the universe.

- ☥ *Affirm Today*: Today I live in the realm of the spiritual masters. My body is my servant, its habits, addictions, cravings and desires have no control over my spiritual power. I as spirit in physical form choose life.

- ☥ *Affirm Today*: I have been meaning to treat my body temple to a fresh meal prepared by my own loving hands.

- ☥ To heal requires an unconditional commitment to living your best self and encouraging the same in others. Affirm: I am seeking perfect health.

- ☥ To eat in the spirit of nourishment for perfect health I affirm: All food I eat and prepare for my loved ones is a reflection of the care I honor for myself and their life of longevity.

Meditation

The essential nature of man is peace. Meditation is a spiritual tool used for bringing balance to all aspects of life. Meditation enriches the spirit, mind, body and emotions. Meditation as a spiritual tool will calm most anxiety, clear the mind and balance the heart rate. Using meditation as a detox therapy involves teaching the client breathing techniques to create a calm spirit. Any form of spiritual development always begins with nurturing the breath. There are more than twenty-five popular types of breath techniques used in meditation, yoga and relaxation therapy. It is recommended that you begin to expand your knowledge to be able to work with the learning styles of your various clients. There are a multitude of programs to learn breathing and meditation so please take the time to research these if you need to increase your knowledge as a therapist enabling your comfort in teaching meditation sessions.

Some additional first steps for using meditation is to learn how to sit and to keep the eyes closed. This helps to focus the mind to begin the art of concentration. This is achieved by repeating a positive affirmation in the mind. Once your client becomes more aware of themselves on a spiritual level you may have them to begin visualizations such as seeing themselves in nature and seeing their body cleansed and free from disease. A series of visualizations can always assist the body in its detoxification process.

The mind is very powerful in the healing process. If a person thinks they are sick or in fear of dying from a disease diagnosis, this thinking becomes a part of the cellular memory. The cells of the body have the ability to do exactly what our internal energy tells them to do. It is always better to think positive in the face of health challenges. Thoughts are constant affirmations that direct the body and it is far better to say, "Today I'm living in peace, love and good health." This tells the cells to help you feel better every day. Some of the benefits of meditation include:

- ◊ Increases blood flow
- ◊ Slows the heart rate
- ◊ Leads to a deeper level of physical relaxation
- ◊ Good for people with high blood pressure
- ◊ Decreases muscle tension
- ◊ Helps in chronic diseases
- ◊ Enhances the immune system
- ◊ Reduces emotional distress
- ◊ Enhances energy
- ◊ Helps with weight loss
- ◊ Improves air flow to the lungs
- ◊ Decreases the aging process
- ◊ Cures headaches and migraines
- ◊ Normalizes weight
- ◊ Harmonizes the endocrine system
- ◊ Relaxes the nervous system
- ◊ Beneficial for brain electrical activity
- ◊ Builds self-confidence
- ◊ Resolves phobias and fears
- ◊ Helps control negative thoughts
- ◊ Helps with focus and concentration
- ◊ Increases creativity
- ◊ Improves learning ability and memory
- ◊ Increases feelings of vitality and rejuvenation
- ◊ Increases emotional stability
- ◊ Improves relationships
- ◊ Makes it easier to remove bad habits

- ◊ Improves relations at home and work
- ◊ Develops will power
- ◊ Helps in quitting smoking, alcohol addiction
- ◊ Reduces dependency on drugs and pharmaceuticals
- ◊ Helps cure insomnia
- ◊ Develops emotional maturity
- ◊ Provides peace of mind, happiness
- ◊ Brings body, mind, spirit in harmony
- ◊ Changes attitude toward life

A meditation session can begin either before or after the opening of the client's appointment time. Sit down with your client with some relaxing music playing and instruct them to begin to breathe deeply, such as with abdominal breathing for up to 5 minutes depending on the client's experience.

Chakra Therapy Detox

The chakras are energy centers in the aura that regulate the energy entering and flowing throughout the physical and energy bodies. The life force is channeled to the physical body through the chakras. Often a client will need energetic cleansing from the high levels of stress and negative energy that they encounter. Chakras allow for easy assessment of a person's energetic body. Reading chakras are done with a pendulum or through chakra scanning. The intention here is not to explain the working of each chakra but to inform you as a future therapist that learning chakra therapy is an excellent skill that is beneficial to every client. Most times when you become certified in other energy healing methods, chakra therapy is always included.

The point of Chakra Therapy Detox is to use different vibrations of sound and energy to help open and balance the continuous flow of energy to the body for health maintenance. The energy flow of each chakra can be interrupted by social issues, ailments, low vibrations, stress or anything that a person encounters that does not support their purpose or respect their divinity. This broad range of negative forces that are prevalent in the world today permeates the existence of most mentally and emotionally immature people who have not learned to spiritually fortify themselves. Unfortunately, this may be every client that you treat.

The Techniques of Chakra Therapy Detox include:
Naturopathic Reiki Therapy (see section on Touch Therapy)

Crystal Therapy: uses the energy of crystals to align vibrational frequencies and draw out energetic debris. The use of crystal grids is very effective for unblocking the chakras and administering penetrating cellular equalizers for the human form. Wand and pendulum work is for both cleansing and energizing the chakras. These specially formed crystals are activators of concentrated energy based on the type, color and density of the crystal material. Highly dense wands and crystals align themselves energetically with the upper chakras, for example lapis lazuli or diamonds. Medium density crystals such as all types of quartz, agates and calcites are flushing crystals that remove energy debris from the middle and lower chakras. Medium density crystals also replace a supply of pure toned energy into the spaces where negative energy is extracted from.

Color Therapy Infusion affects the body's internal systems that correlate to each chakra, which creates positive vibrational effects on the client's mood, and present illness, and energizes the internal organs. It is done through color visualization, using color light therapy sessions, eating food of specific colors and wearing the prescribed color.

Vibration Therapy is music or definitive sounds used to promote enlightenment, healing, relaxation, and physical well-being. The musical notes affect the body and organs. High vibrations stimulate the mind and brain functions to make better decisions. Enhance with high pitched jazz, nature sounds, flute and classical music. Middle tones affect the mid sections of the body, such as the heart, lungs, stomach, etc. Enhance with jazz, R&B, Reggae, and blues songs. The lower tones stimulate the lower extremities and reproductive systems. Enhance with drum music, such as African, Native American, Kahuna drums, etc.

Tones:
- Low C – Colon and reproductive cleanse
- D – Digestive cleanse
- E – Renewing the vital organs
- F – Cleansing the blood
- G – Eliminating negativity
- A – Making better decisions
- B – Thought pattern changes
- High C – Brain stimulation for overall body, mind and spirit nourishment

Pranic Healing is a detoxing and cleansing technique for the chakras, the auras and the overall health of the body, mind and soul. It uses energetic sweeping for cleansing and energizing in a hands-off method that rebuilds depleted areas and dissipates congestion in the chakras. It is a complete healing system in and of itself and excellent for Chakra Detox Therapy.

Elemental Therapy is the use of the elements that are aligned with each chakra as an additional sublunary method of detoxing and healing the chakras and the body. The elements of air, fire, water, earth and spirit are used in therapy to reconnect the body, aura and chakras with its natural essence by bringing the body directly in touch with the physical properties of the elements.

Food Therapy involves the response of each chakra to the energies of nutrients that includes eating specific foods that affect the flow of the chakras. In chakra food therapy clients are coached on consuming foods that will intensify the vibration of their chakra where blockages, congestion and dirty energy has manifested. Included in food therapy is also the consumption of herbs that add nutrition and medicinal value to balancing out the causes of the chakra imbalances.

Essential Oils Therapy is also considered an additional herbal therapy because of the high concentration of the herbal, nutritional and medicinal content in the organic therapeutic grade oils that are used for health regimens. Just like with the plants that are consumed for food, the chakras are paired with plant properties that have proven to have positive regenerating effects therefore, there are several different oils that can be used with each chakra depending on the needs of the client.

Chakra Breathing techniques are a series of breath works that increase frequency of the energy flowing through the chakras. Each breath in aligned with the physical location of the chakra and raises the energetic output of the chakra.

Meditation and Visualization Therapy for chakras is a soothing method of enhancing the work the chakras do for the body. To visualize cleansing and good health is beneficial for every cell in the body. This technique is best for reprogramming the cellular function of the body to reflect health and wellness. Meditation for beginners is quiet guided listening, learning to chant, learning to release thought processes to enter a realm of peaceful existence, and participating in quiet guided visualization as a mindful manifestation that helps the meditator gain inner awareness to assist with changing or creating something powerful, usually for short periods of time. More advanced clients can have lengthier meditation therapies that open portals of knowledge to assist with their healing.

Some of these therapies do require advanced training to learn them effectively and remember only when you have become proficient in these chakra therapies for yourself is when you can effectively share this health therapy with your clients.

When chakra therapy detox is successful the client will begin to see actual changes in their energy body, their attitude about living in good health and their commitment to maintaining consistency for longevity.

Chapter 8 Sample Detox Programs

Detoxification is a gradual process that can be as little as a seven-day cleanse to a few years depending on what your client wants to change. Set small attainable goals and give your clients daily reminders of the goals they have set for their health. A system of consistent detoxification should be an annual part of a healthy person's lifestyle routine.

The formulation of a Detox Care Plan is based on the results of the client's assessment. Which includes an intake form, client interview on their health needs, an analysis of their eating lifestyle, facial analysis, pH analysis and urine analysis. The results of which will assist you in determining the recommended length of the program. In a standard Detox Care Plan the following list serves as a guide to the areas to include:

- Program Dates
- Cleansing Regimen
- Meal Plan or Restaurant Suggestions
- Herbal Plan (optional)
- Detox Therapy Schedule
- Follow up appointment

Sample Detox Program-21 DAYS

Eliminate all processed foods, sugar, dairy, meat and seafood

Begin with the Natural Foods Detox Formula for 7 days

Eat only live foods for full 21 days
Daily fresh juice of fruits, vegetables and greens
Provide a menu
Detox herbs or supplements for purging
Develop a system of meditation/affirmations for the client
Encourage your client to reduce their levels of stress
Schedule a Detox therapy at least once a week

There are many variations available for detoxing, each program will be personalized for every client. If you receive any resistance from your client, encourage them to remember why they are trying to change their health and to keep their vision of health in mind.

Create a Detox Maintenance Profile for each of your clients. This checklist will make it easy to compile the Detox Care Plan and serves as a quick view for referencing the plan.

What happens after the detox is over? Detox lifestyle plan is put together with the client as suggestions on what they can permanently do to maintain the health benefits from the regular detox.

- Develop a non-toxic home environment
- Do a kitchen makeover to preserve health
- Use filters or natural water system in the home
- Switch to natural fiber clothing
- Use natural cleaning products

Case Studies

The following are case studies from certified Detox Therapists and Detox Care Programs they formulated. Although every detox program is unique, let these serve as examples to assist with your professional formulas.

7 Day Detox

Detox Assessment
Detox Questionnaire Results Summary
Female
Age 35
Client smokes cigarettes between 5 and 10 times per day.
She experiences fatigue in the body.
Client's sexual function is decreased.
She sleeps well from 6 to 8 hours.
Eating lifestyle includes meat, processed food, salt in food, and eats out at restaurants occasionally. She drinks at least 8 glasses of water daily.

Client is diagnosed with diabetes and high blood pressure and is currently prescribed and taking lisinopril (for high blood pressure) and glimepiride (for high blood sugar). She states that the doctor says that her illnesses are stable at this time.

She hopes to gain energy, a clear mind, and better eyesight.

Facial analysis:
Client has stress in the circulatory and respiratory

regions of the face. Client has dark rings around eyes, top and bottom, including puffiness and bags underneath eyes which indicates kidney and liver stress. She also has darkness in the bottom of the face near the digestive and reproductive region of the face.

pH testing summary:
5.5 acid

Food Recommendations:
A liquid fast is suggested for at least 3 days. If unable to do so eating all raw fruits and veggies for the first 3 days is recommended, continue with cooked vegan meals thereafter for the next 4 days. After the first 7 days strive to complete 7 more days, and for two more weeks if possible. Eat seasonal and organic food whenever possible. First 7 days should be without salt, and no smoking. Avoid salt to give taste buds a rest and for the best possible results of the regeneration process. Use fresh herbs and seasonings when possible. Food prep can help to stay on track with a busy schedule.

Meal Planning and Herbal detox:
First 3 days: Drink spring water and detox drink throughout your day

1 cup of warm lime water upon rising

Breakfast: 1-2 cups of moringa tea w/2 tablespoons of sea moss

Mid-morning: 1-2 cups of burdock root tea

Lunch: 1-2 cups of burdock root tea including 2 tablespoons of sea moss

Before dinner: 1-2 cups of burdock root tea

Dinner: 1 cup of herbal tea of choice and 1 cup of warm lime water

Next 4 days: Drink ½ gallon spring water per day, remembering to not drink and eat at the same time. Have suggested beverages at least 30-minutes to 1 hour before or after meals of solid foods.

1 cup of warm lime water with 2 tablespoons of sea moss upon rising

Breakfast: green smoothie including moringa tea or fruit of choice

Mid-morning: Salad greens or vegetables of choice
1-2 cups of burdock root tea

Lunch: salad w/lime juice, 1 fruit
1-2 cups of burdock root tea with 2 tablespoons of sea moss or green smoothie with tea and sea moss

Before dinner snack: vegetable of choice
1-2 cups of burdock root tea

Dinner: 1 cup of herbal tea of choice and 1 cup of warm lime water

Herbal therapy:
Sea moss 2-3 times daily provides minerals needed and can curb appetite.

Elderberry 2-3 times daily as a detoxifier.

Burdock root-2-3 times daily as a detoxifier and appetite suppressant.

Moringa can be drank all throughout day to curb coffee cravings and free radical eliminator.

St John's Wort 1 time daily if feeling anxious or to relax after work.

Damiana leaf 1 time daily or every other day to stimulate libido.

These herbs are to be consumed as tea as they are dried and can be brewed. Drink elderberry, burdock root, sea moss, and moringa daily. Keep sea moss refrigerated after prepared, it can be taken along with a tea or in smoothies. Moringa can be consumed all throughout the day to curb coffee cravings and as a free radical eliminator. Follow instructions provided on the herbs packaging and prepare ahead of time to stay on track.

Recommended fruits and vegetables:
Vegetables

Kale	Cucumber	Onions
Avocado	Bell peppers	Lettuce
Greens	Okra	Squash
Tomato	Zucchini	

Fruits

Melons	Dates	Berries
Limes	Mangoes	Pears
Cherries	Seeded grapes	

Remember to purchase fresh seasonings and herbs.

Touch therapy:
If possible, take out the time to receive a massage as this can help induce relaxation in order to stay on track in this process. Lymphatic drainage is a highly recommended therapy. If you are unable to receive a lymphatic drainage massage during the detox period, an alternative is to purchase a loofah and mildly scrub body once daily in the morning or before bed. Start from the feet up and brush toward the heart.

Metaphysics and Movement detox recommendations:
Establish a set time of 5 to 20 minutes before starting your day to meditate and write out what needs to be done throughout the day. As the overall detox process is very important, during the process it is vital to get exercise and movement daily to help the toxins to release through sweating, which also helps with mood balancing. If you are unable to join a gym, get a trainer or workout from home, find a park and try to get a jog or run in for at least 30 minutes to 1 hour for a minimum of 3 days throughout the week. Use stairs at work. Also wearing and or visualizing red colors while relaxing can help with energy and sexual power. Use daily affirmations to stay strong in this pivotal journey.

For example, "I am love, I am light, I am peace, I am what I am" or "Just for today: I will not be angry. I will not worry. I will show appreciation. I will work hard on myself. I will be kind to every living thing."

Please call after the first three days.

21 Day Detox

Detox Assessment
Detox Questionnaire Results Summary
Male
Age 29
Facial Analysis Summary:
  Bags under eyes with crows feet (Kidney)
  Slight swelling under bottom lip (Colon)

pH Testing Summary:
  Overall body pH 6.5 Normal

Detox Regimen Components:
  No processed foods
  Natural Foods Detox Formula once daily
  Fresh juice daily
  Herbal supplements
  Therapeutic detoxing
  Touch therapy
  Detox movement
  Metaphysical detoxing

Recommended Herbal Therapies:
  Kava Kava for sleeping
  Casacara Sagrada for constipation

Recommended Supplements:
  E3 Live for protein, vitamin B12 and antioxidants
  Wheatgrass for chlorophyll and minerals

Recommended Touch Therapy:
  Reflexology for deep relaxation, increased circulation and relieve migraine headaches

Recommended Movement Therapy:
Walking to sweat

Recommended Metaphysical Therapies:
Meditation and Affirmations

Meals:
Maintain eating two meals a day with a concentration on adding more vegetables and live foods. When eating out during the detox program commit to ordering a salad before each meal.

Liquid Nourishment Recipes:
Natural Foods Detox Formula
- 4 cups of spring water
- Juice of 1 fresh squeezed lemon
- 1-2 cloves of garlic
- 1-2 shakes of cayenne pepper
- Agave nectar or maple syrup to taste (for additional nutrients) (optional)
- ¼ - ½ cup of organic extra virgin cold pressed olive oil

Juices:
Green Lemonade:
- 1 head of green leaf lettuce
- 1 whole organic lemon
- 5 – 6 stalks of kale
- 1 to 2 organic apple
- optional (1 to 2 tablespoon of fresh ginger)
- Add equal parts water and drink in 8 ounce servings

Green Juice:
- ½ cup of fresh spinach
- 1 small handful of fresh parsley

½ cup of fresh kale
½ cup of cilantro
2 stalks of celery
1 small ginger peeled
1 cucumber chopped
1 cup fresh pineapple
2 tablespoon fresh lemon juice
Add equal parts water and drink in 8 ounce servings

Beet Juice:
1 organic cucumber
1 small beet peeled and chopped
1 small carrot
1 to 2 tablespoon fresh lemon juice
1 small apple (cored & roughly chopped)
Add equal parts water and drink in 8 ounce servings

Cucumber Juice:
3 large stalks celery
1 cucumber
1 large carrot
¼ bunch fresh cilantro
Add equal parts water and drink in 8 ounce servings

Spinach Juice:
2 bunches of fresh spinach leaves
1 medium apple
1 small lime
Add equal parts water and drink in 8 ounce servings

Smoothies:
    Kale Smoothie:
    2 handfuls of kale
    1 avocado
    1 tsp. maca root powder
    ½ - 1 cup of ice
    Add water for desired thickness

    Antioxidant Smoothie:
    1 avocado
    2 figs
    ½ cup blueberries
    ½ tsp. of flaxseeds
    Add water for desired thickness

    Immune Booster Smoothie:
    2 handfuls of spring greens
    1 avocado
    1 cup mango
    ½ lemon juice
    ½ - 1 cup of ice
    Add water for desired thickness

    Protein Smoothie:
    2 handfuls of spring greens
    1 avocado
    ¼ cup of cashews (soaked and rinsed)
    1 cup mango
    ½ - 1 cup ice
    Add water for desired thickness

28 Day Detox
Detox Questionnaire Results Summary:
Client - 31 year old male
No current medical conditions or medications

Taking a multi-vitamin
Wants to detox to raise metabolism to promote weight loss
Already eats some organic foods
Eats meat, dairy and occasionally eats processed foods

pH testing summary:
7.0 Normal

Facial Analysis summary:
Red swollen cheeks
Bumpy and greasy along the eyebrow ridge
Broken capillaries in cheeks and nostrils
Sagging jowls
Swollen outside of lower lip
Dark circles around the eyes
Client has issues with mucus due to dairy and very little physical movement
Insufficient lung function due to little or no exercise
Client has admitted to irregularities in digestion and loose stools
Client has fluctuations in blood pressure; sometimes high, sometimes normal
Client also says urination is fine, however, sometimes he has urges to urinate, but nothing comes out

Touch Therapy:
Reiki once a week. Client has never done Reiki before and was a bit hesitant, however he found the therapy quite soothing. I also played soothing nature sounds.

We also talked about meditation. Says it really helped with clearing his mind and dealing with stress.

Suggested Menu:
Breakfast: fresh fruits in a cup of oatmeal and green juice

Mid-morning snack: a handful of almonds and berries

Lunch: a big colorful salad (non-dairy dressing)

Mid-afternoon snack options: apple with almond butter or cut up celery and carrots

Dinner: wild rice and steamed or raw vegetables
Second option: sautéed eggplant with sweet potatoes and cut up cucumbers dashed with sea salt

Side note, only use organic seasonings and real sea salt to season all foods. Irradiated seasonings will not help you to detox and are not good to consume after your detox protocol is complete.

Detox Care Plan Results:
The client felt better overall. He reported having more energy, is using the bathroom better, less bloating and says he is able to handle stress better. He said he will consider doing this detox again. His face wasn't as puffy and less red.

42 Day Detox
Detox Assessment
Detox Questionnaire Results Summary:
Female
24 years old
Mother of four
The client's biggest area of concern is allergies. Client suffers from a variety of allergies, both food and air

borne. Client is okay now, but has dealt with numerous skin problems in the past which still flare up from time to time. Client's daily diet can be toxic to the skin. Client eats out a lot and consumes soda, candy and processed foods. Client does not consume adequate amounts of water and fresh produce. Although client is physically active and has an exercise regimen, her energy is inconsistent. Client has had stomach troubles in the past.

Facial Analysis Summary:
Client has acne scarring all over face. Face is "rough" in appearance especially in cheek areas where skin is slightly darker than in other areas of the face which indicates respiratory stress. Kidney facial signs show organ weakness, stress and insufficient function.

pH Testing Summary:
Saliva: 6.0 - Urine: 7.0 - Average pH: 6.3
Overall, the client is acid. Possible severe to chronic stress on the kidneys.

The main goal for this 42 day detox is to relieve and support the kidneys, respiratory system and clear the skin.

Detox Regimen Components:
Drink at least 8 cups of water a day. Starting every morning with warm water and lemon for the first 14 days, client does not want the Natural Detox Formula. Client has agreed to consume daily morning power smoothies adding healthy snack foods, such as apples, cucumbers and other fresh produce. Lunch will be the heaviest meal of the day between 11am and 1pm and should include a healthy meal with salad, two

vegetables, a bowl of grains and legumes. Dinner time before 7pm will be light and include a cup of legumes and grains with a light salad or steamed vegetable.

Avoid foods that cause the most common allergy and acne flair ups, such as wheat, soy, citrus, nuts, milk, yeast and processed sugary foods. Eliminate all candy and soda. Foods to focus on include kidney beans, cucumbers, green apples, cantaloupe, cranberries, watermelon, and small amounts of honey. Add parsley, onions, ginger, turmeric, rosemary and garlic as meal seasonings. Client can use a honey mustard and agave mix or olive oil and pink Himalaya salt as a salad dressing on the before meal salad. The following foods list should be purchased weekly for the entire month in addition to a 7 day rotating menu.

Shopping List
Case of natural spring water in convenience bottles
Brown rice
Quinoa
Lentils, kidney beans or preferred bean variety
Green leaf lettuce, romaine lettuce or spring salad mix
Parsley, red onion, garlic buds, ginger root, rosemary
Cucumber, green apples, cantaloupe, dried cranberries, watermelon, bell peppers, tomatoes, carrots, cabbage, celery, avocado
Frozen smoothie fruit: mangoes, cherries, peaches, and blueberries
3 fresh young coconuts
Plant-based protein powder of choice
Honey, agave or maple syrup

7 Day Rotating Menu

>Breakfast: Lemon water, Power Smoothie or grain granola, fruit

>Lunch: Salad choice, bean and grain choice, 2 vegetable choices

>Dinner: salad or vegetable choice, cup of legumes and or grain choice, or a smoothie as the meal substitute

Choose a multivitamin with Vitamin A, Vitamin B5, Vitamin C, Bioflavonoids, Vitamin E, and Zinc. Client purchased the plant based multivitamin 4PG from our available stock of New Body Products.

Recommended Herbal Therapy:
Burdock, 2 capsules during the day for skin and blood cleansing

Bee pollen, 2 capsules with breakfast for energy boost

2 dandelion and 2 CKLS capsules in the evening for purging and regeneration.

Herbs were purchased from our current stock of New Body Products.

Recommended Touch Therapy:
Reflexology and ion foot baths 2-3 times per week. Organic therapy facials once a week with black moor mud or green clay mask, facial steams and peppermint moisturizing mist. No heavy oils on the face.

Ion Foot Baths and reflexology appointments are scheduled for Friday evening and Sunday afternoons. Facial will be included in Sunday sessions.

Metaphysics and Movement Components:
Chakra Healing Therapy, Reiki, Coaching support especially around family issues.

Chakra Healing Naturopathic Reiki session is scheduled for Wednesday evenings one time per week.

Chapter 9 Detox Therapist Business

When you are ready to move into the professional service of Detox Therapy, it will take some planning for your business success. If you have no experience in owning and operating a successful business, please properly prepare for this endeavor by taking a business course. They are available sometimes free of charge at your local chamber of commerce or small business association. In today's marketplace there are also free online business courses too. I have seen so many learn a new wellness therapy and program and they have all the enthusiasm in the world when it is time to opening a business yet they have little to no experience in business, and without coaching or a plan for dedication, they soon fall by the wayside and give up moving on to the next thing in life. However, there is still not enough of this type of service in the country to affect the masses of people who desire a healthier way of living a disease-free life. Most communities need therapists and business owners with a high level of consistency for this natural way of living to help the many people who are suffering because of the ways of the world today.

The first step in Detox Therapy business is working on yourself and possibly your family to "test" out the programs that you want to offer professionally. Setting up your business plan and surveying your market for the services you intend to offer is paramount. Know your business. Detox as a principle and function of wellness is nothing new. Many wellness service providers offer information and programs to their clients. However, a Certified Detox Therapist is a specialization that says you have achieved a level of education that renders you qualified and confident to assist clients in their quest to improve not only their bodies but their lives also. Be able to talk to anyone with a clear understanding of what it is you are offering in products and services.

Starting with the success of the business in mind as part of the initial planning and full development of the following components which are to be included in your written business plan.

Business name
Although it is such an honor to have your business named after yourself, your business name should make it easy for your target market to find you. If you are in a big to medium sized city it might be ideal, if the business name includes the city and the service, for example, The Atlanta Detox Center. This type of name is an easy find for anyone searching for this service in a city of millions of potential clients.

Business Objective
What do you want to accomplish with this business in the community? This must be clearly thought out and articulated for yourself, possibly your staff and most of

all it is a good focal point for building and expanding your business as it grows.

Personal Objective

What does this business mean for you and your life? Again, to articulate this will be a great motivator when things get rough or seem uncertain. To be reminded of why you wanted to start this business will keep you motivated.

Market Research

How are other businesses similar to your area of professional service performing in the current market? Are they struggling or are they prosperous? Avoid using this step to compare yourself to any other business. This evaluation will help you to understand the demand of your market. You can have the best idea, but if the market is not interested you will know this by the success of your predecessors.

Location Research

Location is the key to a successful business. Choosing the one that is right for your business involves a few factors. Make your location convenient for your clients to travel to. Ensure that your costs in renting or leasing space does not exceed 25% of your projected business income.

Often new therapists start small and choose a mobile Detox Therapist Service, where you go to your client's home or office to provide the service. This has become very appealing to many consumers. If you decide to go this route be sure to map out designated travel areas and include travel service costs such as an extra fee for fuel and long distances, insurance and maintenance costs for the vehicle.

The home office is another small business option. A home office holds a lot of advantages: no rental fees or additional mortgage, no travel time to work, and total control over hours of operation. The only possible disadvantage is that it reduces the privacy factor of your home.

Rental office space in a building, shopping center, or an existing clinic may be feasible for your budget. Most rental spaces are rented by the square foot, on a weekly or monthly basis and there are set business hours that you must adhere to. In choosing a location you must do your location research to determine the convenience of the location for your clients and yourself in relationship to your travel time to and from work each day. When renting space in an existing clinic or shop, you must consider what your clients will be exposed to in the surroundings, and you must adhere to any rules set forth by the existing establishment. It is very much like a partnership. Another option for a business location would be ownership. A real estate investment is good for your overall financial portfolio, and if you decide to expand, move, or retire from the business, you will have accumulated some equity for your future endeavors.

Marketing Plan
Marketing is seventy-five percent of what you do in business for the first three years. If no one knows about your business, it will not be successful. A great way to start or launch your business is to use a celebrity face to promote your business by getting in front of their audience. If this is not possible then start your marketing the tried and true way by connecting to the community where your business is located, setting up an online presence, using print media, and getting the word out by mouth.

"What's your website?" That will be one of the first questions you will be asked when talking to others about your business. Your website will be one of your best marketing tools in today's business market. Your website should answer the question: What can you do for me? Vague and secretive websites turn browsers off and they move on. Make your website inviting with a clear and compelling message. Most websites today are do-it-yourself products and very easy to manage. Prices for web hosting are now very affordable and often times free. Start small with a one page site and as your business grows then your website should expand as well. If you do not already have a website, I suggest one of the *free popular sites like Wix, Weebly, Web.com, WordPress, etc.* There are many more, do your research to find which one works best for you. They all have free webpage design platforms that make it easy for you to create and upload for immediate updates. When your website is up and running make sure that it stays up to date with all your current contact information, services, location, and events. It may also be beneficial to have a consultation from a web designer who helps new site users. There are many things to learn like setting up your online payment options, scheduling calendar, mailing list, keywords, metatags and landing page optimization techniques.

Print marketing is newspaper, magazines, postcards, flyers, brochures, and business cards. You need all of these for consistent marketing, especially in your local area. Your business card and brochures are your first form of print marketing. They are offered free or low cost on the internet, and most times you only pay for shipping. Start with a basic business card that gives your name, contact info, website, email, and services. You can make the brochures yourself using Microsoft Word or Publisher programs. Postcards and flyers are optional, however if you are holding classes or events they are a great form of advertising at the hot spots where interested clients are sure to find them. Newspaper and magazine advertisements can be expensive; however, there are free ways of getting in your local and national publications. Most have free community calendars, and take contributing articles from experts in their field. You can also present yourself and your holistic health program as a story of interest and have an article written about you.

Radio, television, and the internet are the electronic media avenues available for business marketing. Let's start with the easy one first, the internet. You can advertise on the internet with social media, banners, links, free business listings, internet radio shows and ads, internet television, and webinars. It is vital to take the time or hire a professional to research and put together a package for you that will tap each one of these areas to potentially broaden your marketing reach.

Marketing only works if there is a consistent effort. Three forms of marketing a day should be a regular part of your business strategy. Use every opportunity for marketing in all forms. Embrace those strategies that work and weed out those strategies that don't. A marketing assistant is a good job for that willing worker that volunteers their time to help your efforts. Don't wait too long to measure your marketing efforts for you need to know very shortly into the endeavor if it is beneficial for your business or not. If not don't be afraid to save time and money by eliminating the failing marketing activity after a set amount of time. Remember also that developing marketing partnerships are a great way to share the expense of marketing. Link up with your affiliates to do some of the more expensive forms of advertising.

Operations Coordination

This portion of the business is where you decide your standard operating procedures, coordinate your staff or your schedule for running the business. Operations areas to consider include, but are not limited to type of business registration, intake consultation forms, documentation forms, a disclaimer statement, fees, products, hours, services and finances.

Employment as a Detox Therapist

A Certified Detox Therapist is also an employable profession. There are spas, health centers, gyms, naturopath offices, chiropractic clinics and more that are looking for qualified personnel with detoxification training.

Detox Therapy business will be hard work, but you are encouraged to plan well with the success of your business always in the forefront of your mind. All wellness modalities are needed in all communities. Detoxing will never go away because people will always be interested in obtaining and maintaining their good health.

Acknowledgements

When wellness becomes a way of life it is second nature to do the things that are healthy for the body, mind and spirit. It can be described as living with a consciousness of balance that is constantly keeping the scales of good health equal, especially in a world where there are many involuntary factors that are operating against good health daily.

The Detox Therapist Course at A Life Of Peace Wellness Education Institute was developed to provide a unique wellness professional to the community that not only works with the physical components of detoxification, but also the mental, emotional and spiritual deficiencies that make many unhealthy lifestyles permanent. For more than eleven years I have worked with clients and students who have committed to changing their lifestyles and have accredited that change to their initial detoxification program and care plan. It is to these many individuals who have inspired my work, research, learning and dedication to the regenerative magnificence of the detoxification process that I acknowledge as the source of inspiration for this book.

As always in every endeavor of my life I give thanks to my number one photographer, supporter and love of my life story Dr. Chenu Gray. My sons Kazembe, Jajah and Bomani Gray as a great source of support that I can rely on without fail. A special thank you to Fayola Herod "the editor" that I trust completely with her expertise and insight for the entire A Life Of Peace Wellness Therapy Series. I also want to thank myself for being open to the life works that chose me as a vessel of love, light, peace and progress to the world community.

About the Author

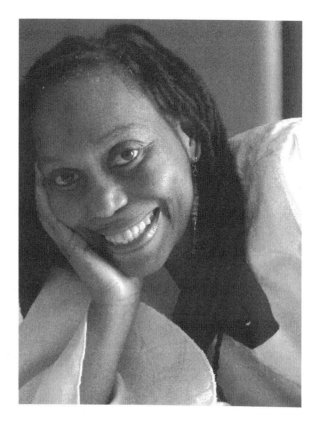

K. Akua Gray is the author of ten published works in holistic health and vegan nutrition. As the primary curriculum developer for A Life Of Peace Wellness Education Institute and naturopath instructor, Akua has been writing on health and wellness for over two decades. Born in Houston, TX, K. Akua Gray now lives in Ghana, West Africa.

References

Afua, Queen (2012) <u>Heal Thyself for Health and Longevity</u>. Hunlock Creek PA: E World Publishing, Inc.

Batmanghelidj, M.D., F. (2001) <u>Your Body's Many Cries for Water</u>. Vienna, VA: Global Health Solutions, Inc.

Goss, Dr. Paul. (1995) <u>The Rebirth of the Gods</u>. Compton, CA: D. P. G.

Gray, K. Akua (2016) <u>Natural Health and Wellness: The Consultant Manual</u>. Missouri City, TX: BJK Publishing

Gray, K. Akua (2010) <u>Veggie Delights: Eating Live for Maximum Nutrition and Wellness</u>. Missouri City, TX: BJK Publishing

Ehret, Professor Arnold (1994) <u>The Mucusless Diet Healing System: Scientific Method of Eating Your Way to Health</u>. Ardsley, NY: Ehret Literature Publishing Company

Hass, M.D., Elson M. (1981) <u>Staying Healthy with the Seasons</u>. Berkeley, CA: Celestial Arts

Hass, M.D., Elson M. (2004) <u>The New Detox Diet: The Complete Guide for Lifelong Vitality with Recipes, Menus, & Detox Plans</u>. Berkeley, CA: Celestial Arts

Hyman, M.D., Mark (2008) <u>Ultrametabolism: The Simple Plan for Automatic Weight Loss</u>. New York, NY:

Books

Rose, Natalia (2006) <u>The Raw Food Detox Diet: The Five-Step Plan for Vibrant Health and Maximum Weight Loss</u>. New York, NY: Harper Collins Publishers, Inc.

Rose, Sara (2005) <u>Detox: The Process of Cleansing and Restoration</u>. Bath, UK: Parragon Publishing

Whitaker, N.D., Dr. Scott and Fleming, CN, MH, Jose (2007) <u>Medisin: The Cause & Solutions to Disease, Malnutrition and the Medical Sins that are Killing the World</u>. Wildamor, CA: Divine Protection Publications

Made in the USA
Middletown, DE
08 January 2023